THEN AND NOW

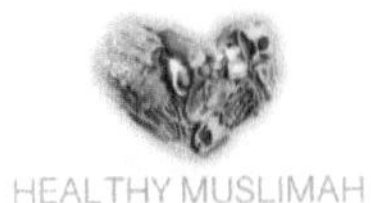

BROUGHT TO YOU BY HEALTHY MUSLIMAH

THEN AND NOW

FOOD IN THE TIME OF THE PROPHET ﷺ AND FOOD NOW

KATE HEPBURN

BBA, Nutrition Consultant

2nd Edition

Notice of Liability

Inquiries may be sent to: info@healthymuslimah.com

1st Printing – February 2019, 2nd Printing - December 2020

Author: Kate Hepburn, BBA, NC

Editor: Um Yusef Jamie Snyder

Disclaimer

ACKNOWLEDGEMENT AND THANKS

Alhamdullilah (All Praise and Thanks are for Allah, the Only True God) Words fail to describe how immensely grateful I am to have the opportunity to share this book with you, remembering that everything comes from Allah, all thanks and praise belong to Allah and any good contained in this book or produced out of it is from Allah alone. Any shortcomings are my own, and I seek forgiveness.

I pray that this book is a means of benefit to everyone who reads it and that Allah accepts it as a small effort towards helping current and future generations around the world gain greater health and wellness for His sake, using time and health to do good and worship Allah to the best of their ability, ameen.

Thank You

The Prophet ﷺ said: "He who does not thank the people is not thankful to Allah." (Sunan Abu Dawud; Sahih according to Al-Albani)[1]

Few people truly understand how much goes into writing a book – the blood, sweat and tears, the worry, the doubts, the time, the cost – and few know how each book writing journey is filled with so many people who made it all possible, each a gift from Allah and each contributing in his or her own special way.

I know my words can never fully capture the journey, nor my immense gratitude to the people who have been such an important part of my life over the years and through this book writing process, nor my gratitude to Allah for sending those people my way. Yet, I hope that my prayers for each of them are answered.

To all the people in my life who have helped make this possible, *thank you.*

I would like to extend special thanks to my parents. In asking Allah to help me thank them, I cannot find better words than those He has given us. Allah addresses all adults in verse 17:24 of the Quran with a beautiful command:

> *"And lower to them the wing of humility out of mercy and say,
> 'My Lord, have mercy upon them as they brought me up [when I
> was] small.'"(Quran 17:24)*[2]

They have spent on me in every way that it is possible to spend, with their effort, care, time, money, hope. They have cared for me even before my first breath, so I ask Allah to support me in never failing to be grateful to them even after my last breath.

FOREWORD

As I was setting out to write this book, I found myself thinking, how on earth do I share this information, which I have gathered over several years, in a way that will not be so depressing and overwhelming that it paralyzes readers and achieves exactly the opposite of what I intend? Admittedly, the thought also crossed my mind several times that readers may hate me after reading this book. I am volunteering myself as the messenger of bad news, and we all know what happens to the messenger.

I still remember exactly the feeling I had upon first discovering the corruption of our food system, and I remember the frustration and distress of not knowing how to approach it, how to navigate the overwhelming amount and extent of information and – quite critically – what to eat! I was miserable. The more I learned, the more stressful things became. I had delved in alone with no one to guide me or offer practical support. I did not know how to make solid or beneficial changes and began bouncing between health food fads – going gluten free, juicing, trying raw food. I was all over the place, and every time I tried something new, I found myself having to learn an entire new way of selecting and preparing food. I would not recommend my trial-and-error approach to anyone, yet I expect there are numerous people in my shoes, who either want to improve their eating habits or at least think they should, and that is what lead me to study nutrition and start Healthy Muslimah. Although exploring and scaling this mountain has certainly not been an easy route, I sincerely believe that the information I have gathered is too important not to share and that many of us are eating food that is robbing us of health and energy without our realizing it. From the start of my health journey, which coincided almost exactly with my conversion to Islam, I have felt that passing this information on is an amaanah, and I am grateful for the opportunity to fulfil that trust by sharing this book with you.

My aim is not to deliver bad news. Discovering the truth about our food is uncomfortable, it is stressful, and it is depressing, but knowing what is going on is not the end goal. It is merely a stepping stone. Knowing, understanding and asking questions are the tools that ultimately enable us to make better choices.

My aim is also not to tell you what you should do or to sit in judgement of your choices. My own choices regarding food have ranged in the past from ordinary to dismal; it was my digestion of loads of information that motivated me to alter my choices. I suspect that such information may resonate with many people and may perhaps spark a desire to make solid changes. In sharing stories of our food system – including dramas, mysteries and certainly some horror – and the effect it is having on our health and the planet, I aim to shed light on options and present possibilities, complete with a vision for health and hope for the future.

The goal of this book is to orient you not with a massive problem but with a solution: to SIMPLIFY healthy eating by getting back to basics. The key to health is not in following fad diets or food gurus but in getting back to eating whole natural food the way Allah made it and the way the Prophet ﷺ ate it. This key opens the door to connecting our food choices to our desire to please our Creator and to taking care of the body with which He has blessed us. Such efforts elevate our choices regarding food to acts of worship.

This is a book about showing you that it's possible. Real health, energy and vitality are within your reach through nourishing your body. It is about presenting a way through the clutter and overwhelm of information and showing you that you have everything to gain by making positive changes, one small step at a time. Simplifying healthy eating and healthy living is at the heart of everything I believe in and everything I do. It is the foundation of Healthy Muslimah, the food philosophy behind this book, and it is why I create programs that are simple and easy to follow. I want to give you what I wish I had when I started out my health journey, which I believe would have made everything so much easier:

> *Breathe. Relax. The key to health is eating natural whole food the way Allah made it in small portions. Take it step by step, be easy with yourself (and others) and start with 'bismillah'.*

Change does not happen overnight. It takes time and may always remain a work in progress. I would love to say that I eat perfectly healthy organic food 100% of the time, but I live in the same food environment as you, and the challenges are real. While this book aims to give you a path to greater health, I also aim to acknowledge our inherent imperfection, particularly my imperfection. My life, my diet and my choices are a work in progress just like everyone's. I pray that you benefit from my experiences and the information I share and want you to know that every goal you set and pursue motivates me further toward mine. Thank you!

> *O Allah, make me better than what they think of me, and forgive me for what they do not know about me, and do not take me to account for what they say about me. (Du'a of Abu Bakr)[3]*

The more we practice, the better we become. We cannot avoid challenges and obstacles that knock us off track. Still, choosing to nourish our bodies, to eat for the sake of taking care of the body Allah has blessed us with and to choose wholesome food means that we are in a better physical state to manage those ups and downs when they arise. Some might think nutrition consultants exist on a health food pedestal where good choices and changes in habit come easy; that is why sprinkled throughout the book is amazing evidence from ordinary sisters who have made changes themselves and felt the benefits. People just like you. The amazing thing is that just knowing it is possible changes everything.

But don't take my word for it. Read on and see for yourself.

And as you go, remember to…

Breathe. Relax. The key to health is eating natural whole food the way Allah made it in small portions. Take it step by step, be easy with yourself (and others) and start with 'bismillah'.

Table of Contents

Acknowledgements and Thanks

Foreword

PART ONE: THE ROOT OF THE PROBLEM
Duped, 15
A Vision of Health and Hope, 33
Abundance and Excess, 39
Just One Third, 46
Then and Now: An Overview, 59

PART TWO: A CORRUPTED FOOD SUPPLY
Processed Food, 63
Additives, 64
Pesticides, 71
Genetically Modified Food, 79
Nutrient Density, 85

PART THREE: FOOD, THEN AND NOW
Sugar, 88
Honey, 93
Artificial Sweeteners, 95
Grains, 98
Oil and Fats, 103
Milk and Dairy, 109

Meat, 112
Chicken, 118
Eggs, 123
Fish and Seafood, 129
Water, 131
Packaging and Cooking, 135

PART FOUR: FOOD, HEALTH, HEALING AND HOPE
Total Load: The Sum of the Parts, 139
Gut Health, 145
The Creator Knows What the Creation Needs, 151
Our Body Has Been Entrusted to Us, 162
How the Prophet ﷺ Ate, 172

PART FIVE: MAKING CHANGES
Foundations for Change, 190
Health Coaching Personal Assessments, 210
Whole Food Shopping List, 221
Beginner's Guide to Navigating Labels, 224
Whole Food Action Plan, 227

PART SIX: A CHALLENGE
The Final Challenge, 230

NOTES, 232

BIBLIOGRAPHY, 247

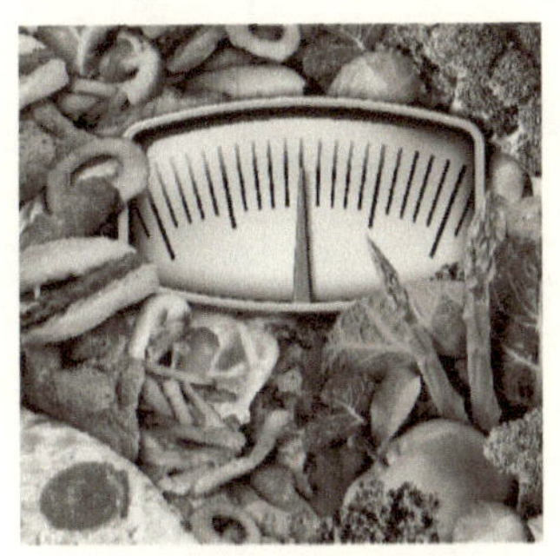

PART ONE
THE ROOT OF
THE PROBLEM

And I will mislead them. (Quran 14:119)

*Eat and drink, but be not excessive. Indeed, He likes
not those who commit excess. (Quran 7:31)*

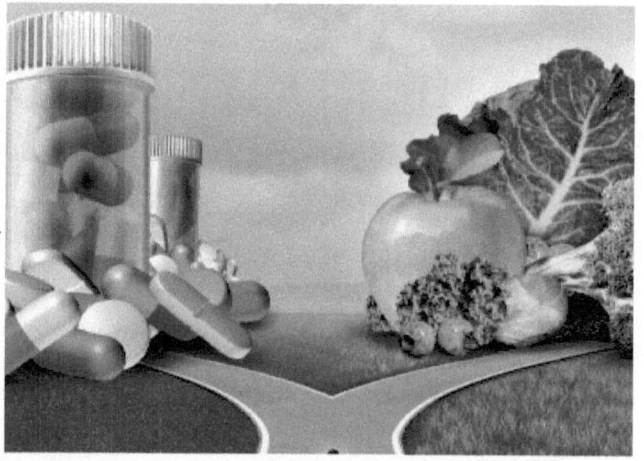

Chapter 1

Duped

As she packed her bag, getting ready to leave for the weekend workshop, she couldn't help but feel a sense of relief. Finally, someone would be able to help. Despite all her hard work, her son was struggling so much with his weight and his health. She had been carefully choosing low fat food and encouraging him to exercise. There were no more sweets or junk foods in the house, but it didn't seem to be making a difference. No matter what she did, it didn't seem to work. The upcoming week-long health camp was the blessing she had been hoping for; when it turned up out of nowhere, she had jumped at the opportunity. Finally, someone was going to support her efforts and get to the bottom of whatever was going on. She could already feel the deadweight lifting from her chest, though she couldn't yet manage a deep breath. Maybe there were underlying issues. Was it genetic? Did he have some sort of illness? She felt a flurry of worry inside her as deep as her womb.

She and her son arrived at the camp along with several other moms and kids who were suffering the same issues. The awkwardness of meeting new people was soon broken by smiles and hellos and a realization that everyone was in the same boat. Nerves, hope and anticipation filled the air as attendees were orientated and told how the weekend camp would run. Once everyone was settled, the first thing on the agenda was for each mom to go through the details of her child's diet with a nutrition specialist, followed by a weigh in and a series of medical checkups, with the first class and a set of sporting activities to begin at 11 am. The nutrition specialists would meet with moms later that afternoon to discuss their initial findings.

Her follow-up appointment was the first on the list at 4 pm. The day flashed by, with moms and kids being shuffled between sports activities, and at 3:50 pm, she was already outside the consultation room. Hope mixed with trepidation flitted in her stomach, and her mouth felt dry. Finally, she was going to have the answer. She'd know what was going on and what she could do. She prayed for a smooth route to her son's improved health. The consultant smiled as she called her in, which allowed her to at least unclasp her hands as she sat down, trying not to look as nervous as she felt. The consultant opened up her folder and started talking matter-of-factly, explaining the findings. Listening intently, her face froze for a moment, then it crumpled as the full impact of the words hit her. She broke down, her hands covering her face, and she sobbed. There was nothing at all medically or genetically wrong with her son. The single reason for his overweight and poor health was the food he'd been eating at home.[4]

DECEIVED BY THE FOOD INDUSTRY

The food industry is big business, and the food we eat has changed dramatically in the last 100 years. Before the commercialization of food, for thousands of years, traditional cultures across the world ate natural whole foods. Even a few hundred years ago, our great grandmas were cooking and eating natural food. This is no longer the case. Our food has been changed, and the way we consume it has changed. In its place, as part of our stress-filled, overwhelmed lives, we are eating a lot of ready-made, commercially-produced food. It is so common, and so unfortunate, that it has come to be known as the SAD diet – the Standard American Diet. We have normalized a new way of eating that is high in refined, processed food as well as fat, sugar, salt and calories while being low in necessary nutrients. It's not limited to fast food; homemade food is increasingly prepared with half-baked convenience products, and even fresh produce comes covered in additives and pesticides. It's also not limited to the US; this wave of highly processed, high sugar, low nutrient food has reached so many parts of the world that SMD – Standard Modern Diet – is a more relevant acronym.

This SMD has replaced traditional natural whole foods with cheap food-like products that are largely designed in a lab to look better, taste better and last longer, and this has had a devastating effect on our health. We all have family or friends with cardiovascular disease and diabetes. We hear of new cases of cancer in our community all the time, and they are increasing. Brothers and sisters are struggling with infertility, with IVF clinics popping up like mushrooms in every town. Children are now developing Type 2 Diabetes, a disease formerly known as adult-onset diabetes because it only affected adults. At the root of so many of these illnesses is *our food*. If we look to nature, animals don't eat natural food to the point of obesity or sickness. Nobody *wants* to get sick, and nobody would actively try to make themselves sick through food choice, yet we have seen a steady rise in food-related disease. It's logical to assume that there is more to our overeating, and our poor food choices, than meets the eye.

To better understand what is going on and how we got here, we first need to step back in time to a period after the Industrial Revolution when a shift in how business was done and how products were promoted changed the world as people knew it. At that moment in history, mass production was in full swing, but producers were concerned: would there come a point when consumers would just stop buying products because they had everything they needed?[5]

The idea of not having something more to buy, not having an 'I want' list, might be a totally foreign concept to most of us. There's always something we are dreaming of purchasing: a new flavor, a new color, a new style, an upgrade. There's an endless variety of enticing goodies to add to our ever-growing collection of stuff. Not wanting to buy more is a concept hard to imagine in our modern consumer environment. However, as far-fetched as it may seem to us, there was a point in history, not all that long ago, when ordinary consumers were much more utilitarian in their shopping choices; they bought products for functional and practical use. Also, up to that point, most products were advertised in functional terms, with a simple focus on a product's virtue such as durability and practical usefulness. Realizing that utilitarian consumers would eventually stop buying more, producers saw that to keep their customers, they would have to change their strategy. To sell more, it would be necessary to make people want more, and to do that, consumers would have to be trained to follow their desires rather than to simply fulfill their needs.[6]

Needs to Desires

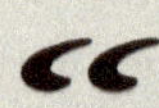

We must shift America from a needs to a desires culture… People must be trained to desire, to want new things even before the old had been entirely consumed. We must shape a new mentality in America. Man's desires must overshadow his needs. (Paul Mazur, Lehman Brothers) [7]

A NEW TYPE OF CONSUMER IS BORN

The man at the center of the new consumer movement, whose influence has seeped into every corner of our lives is probably someone you've never even heard of. Edward Bernays, known as the father of Public Relations, was the nephew of Sigmund Freud. Heavily influenced by his uncle's work, and having understood that people are "rarely aware of the real reasons which motivate their actions,"[8] Bernays began experimenting with novel ways to apply psychological principles. His career took off during World War I, when he had the chance to test propaganda techniques as part of Woodrow Wilson's presidential campaign. The response was astounding. He wondered if the same methods of persuasion could be used during times of peace. Of course, nobody liked the word 'propaganda', so he coined the phrase 'public relations', and a whole new brand of influence was born, one that would be applied to both the public and private sector in years to come and that would play a pivotal role in the development of the fields we now know as public relations, marketing, branding and advertising.[9]

> **❝** *If we understand the mechanisms and motives of the group mind, it is now possible to control and regiment the masses according to our will without their knowing it. In almost every act of our daily lives, whether in the sphere of politics or business, in our social conduct or our ethical thinking, we are dominated by the relatively small number of persons who understand the mental processes and social patterns of the masses. It is they who pull the wires which control the public mind. (Edward Bernays, Propaganda)*[10]

At the time, advertising was mostly focused on selling the functional value of products, but Bernays came up with the idea that you could make people want things they didn't need by linking mass produced goods to their unconscious desires. Bernays simply applied to commerce and industry the propaganda techniques he had used so effectively in politics – with overwhelming results. One of his most astonishing success stories was his campaign to increase cigarette sales to women at a time when female smokers were taboo. Bernays knew that to boost sales to women, he would have to shift public opinion first. To do this, he orchestrated a campaign in which he had rich female socialites hide cigarettes in their clothes and then strategically whip them out and light up during an Easter Sunday parade, ensuring the media caught them on camera. He had alerted the media in advance that these women would be staging a public protest and dubbed the cigarettes 'Torches of Freedom', effectively linking cigarettes to the women's liberation movement and making them a symbol of women's aspirations for a better life and 'equality with men'. Overnight, an established social taboo was obliterated, and the social perception of women smoking transformed to become not just desirable but pro-social, making the idea that women shouldn't smoke anti-social and discriminatory. The campaign went viral, and cigarette sales to women rose and rose. This manifestation of the idea that consent could be engineered and that it was possible to make people behave irrationally if you linked products to their emotions and feelings changed the face of marketing and advertising and opened the flood gates of social engineering for the mere sake of corporate profit.[11]

Business was to change forever after. "Modern business," Bernays proclaimed, "must have its finger continuously on the public pulse. It must understand the changes in the public mind and be prepared to interpret itself fairly and eloquently to changing opinion."[12] Yet, he did not expect public opinion to be the driving force of sales. Rather, the needs of industries would drive public opinion, including public opinion about individual needs. Wants would become needs at the hands of modern business.

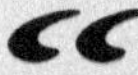

A single factory, potentially capable of supplying a whole continent with its particular product, cannot afford to wait until the public asks for its product; it must maintain constant touch, through advertising and propaganda, with the vast public in order to assure itself the continuous demand which alone will make its costly plant profitable. (Edward Bernays, Propaganda)[13]

CHANGE THROUGH MASS MEDIA

Just as Bernays used socialites, a clever catch phrase and the media to boost cigarette sales, similar mass campaigns have been run since then to influence the public, change perceptions and encourage action, often on an enormous scale, with the force of a social tsunami, and with incredible results. The technique of using television and soap operas to influence society was discovered accidentally in 1969 through a Peruvian TV soap opera called *Simplemente Maria* that told a rags-to-riches story of a young migrant, Maria. The soap covered themes such as class conflict, marriage between rich and poor, the liberation of women, with Maria achieving socio-economic success through her skill in using a Singer sewing machine. Incidentally, sales of Singer machines increased sharply everywhere Maria was watched in Latin America.[14]

Mass media has not only been effective in increasing sales for large companies. Inspired in the 1970s by *Simplemente Maria*, Mexican TV producer Miguel Sabido designed a soap opera to promote adult literacy. *Ven Conmigo (Come with Me)* ran only one year, from 1975-1976, but led to around 1 million illiterates enrolling in adult education classes, an increase of 63% over the previous year. This technique has come to be known as the 'Sabido Effect' and has been widely implemented in countries across the world.[15]

The success of these campaigns illustrates just how easily the masses are influenced, and while increased literacy is no doubt a noble goal, these same techniques have often been used for significantly less savory ideals. They can influence what we buy, even where increasing sales was not the producer's intention, as in the case of *Simplemente Maria*. Television is a powerful tool that brings ideas into our homes and our – and our children's – heads, and has by now been joined by radio, podcasts and a plethora of social media. Subtle but irresistible social messages are coming to us from every angle and reach us along with millions of others with the mere click of a button.

PREDICTABLY IRRATIONAL

We all love to think of ourselves as rational beings making rational decisions, but as it turns out, we are not quite as rational as we think we are. In fact, quite bizarrely, we are often 'predictably irrational', and sometimes all it takes is a single word to make us comply. In a fascinating study done at Harvard, Ellen Langer set up a scenario to test compliance using various combinations of phrases by an actor trying to cut in line at a photocopier. In the first test scenario, the actor said, "Excuse me, I have 5 pages. May I use the xerox machine?" Sixty percent of people allowed him to cut in. In another scenario, the phrase used was, "Excuse me, I have 5 pages. May I use the xerox machine because I'm in a rush?" In this case, compliance jumped to 94%, which makes rational sense to us. Most of us would be happy to help out someone in a rush, but it's scenario number three where things get interesting: "Excuse me, I have 5 pages. May I use the xerox machine, *because I have to make copies*?" Unbelievably, this entirely non-compelling reason yielded an astounding 93% compliance![16] Langer concluded that the word *because* triggers a set of automatic responses, and in decisions where the stakes are low, we will likely respond automatically without any thought simply upon hearing that word. If they are higher, we may give the answer some more thought, but if *because* is used, even with a hardly-compelling reason, there is a good chance we will comply.

According to Robert Cialdini in his must-read book *Influence: The Psychology of Persuasion*, animal species exhibit 'fixed action patterns', which are regular, blindly-mechanical patterns of behavior that, when activated, occur in pretty much the same way and the same sequence every time.[17] Humans, too, have similar preprogramed behaviors, just as we saw in

Ellen Langer's study. This automatic, stereotypical 'decision making' is common in much that we do and is a necessity in a world where we have so much stimulus and so many decisions to make; it provides a shortcut – and we need shortcuts! Without them, we would have to analyze every single little thing we might do before we do it, and it would be impossible to get anything done. Imagine thinking deeply rationally about every single one of the thousands of items at the grocery store before you could make a decision to buy anything. As more and more stimulus is forced on us, we are feeling more and more overwhelmed. The more overwhelmed we feel, the more we rely on shortcuts, even if what they cut short is our rationality. These automatic behavior patterns are very useful, even essential, but they also leave us particularly vulnerable to anyone who knows how to use them – and abuse them – especially if we are unaware that they even exist.[18] In the wrong hands, these triggers can be used as weapons of mass influence[19] to exploit us into buying things we don't need and even things we wouldn't generally want.

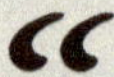

> *There is a group of people who know very well where the weapons of automatic influence lie and who employ them regularly and expertly to get what they want. (Robert Cialdini, Influence, The Power of Persuasion)* [20]

Fixed action patterns, and the automatic triggers that set them off, can be harnessed to persuade us to purchase in the most sophisticated and subtle ways. This phenomenon is why most of us have experienced the situation where we have bought something only to later wonder, why on earth did I buy this? Today's marketers go beyond Bernays' propaganda techniques, relying on key principles to trigger fixed action behavior and prompt us to buy.

These principles – scarcity, social proof, authority, reciprocity, consistency and commitment – can be used individually or in any number of combinations or variations to target each of us personally.[21]

> **Scarcity:** Having something in short supply or at risk of being lost is a very powerful human motivator. When something is

scarce, it becomes valuable. As part of a marketing technique, scarcity is commonly created in the form of limited editions or a sense of urgency with limited spaces or limited time to secure either your seat or special price. We also tend to be happy to pay more for things that we perceive to be rare or limited.

> **Social Proof:** If others are doing it, it must be okay, and if others like it, we will probably like it, too. We use social proof as a shortcut, asking friends what they use, and looking at reviews and starred ratings. Unfortunately, social proof can be engineered. Book authors buy enough copies of their own book to make it a '#1 seller' and to label themselves a best-selling author, (Yes, this is happening even in our communities.) or marketing companies pay women to attend coffee mornings and promote products to other moms, or popular bloggers and vloggers are paid to 'try' products and paid handsomely in return for posting a pic on Instagram, Snapchat, or Facebook. We are particularly inclined to follow social proof from people with whom we identify.

> **Authority**: We have an unsettling reaction to authority, as anyone who is familiar with Stanley Milgram's study on obedience will know. If you're not familiar with it, it's worth spending 20 minutes watching the Milgram study on YouTube to witness a completely irrational level of obedience in the presence of an authority figure. Authority can be established by means of clothing or uniforms, titles or self-proclaimed expertise, all of which are likely to influence us to put our faith in someone claiming to be an expert. In marketing, information, advice and promises issued by an 'authority' can trigger us to blindly follow, which is why so many people swiftly gave up eggs and avocadoes in the past. When 'nutrition authorities' dubbed them unhealthy because of their fat content, we sought refuge in the 'low fat' food industry, which slyly got us hooked on products loaded with sugar and synthetic additives.

> **Liking:** We tend to want to buy from people we like, and what we tend to like most, as humans, are people who are physically

attractive. Seeing someone or something that looks good on the outside triggers a subconscious reaction called the 'halo effect' by which we assume the inside must be good, too. We automatically attribute unrelated and unproven positive qualities to a person that is physically attractive, expecting that they are kind, honest and have a good character. This is why advertisers use actors and models with certain physical features to promote food, clothing, perfume and everything else we buy. We also tend to like people who are similar to us and with whom we identify in personality, opinion, lifestyle and even clothing style. We love to be complimented and consequently like people who compliment us and make us feel good about ourselves. All of these techniques can be rolled into a complex tool designed to influence us to buy.

➤ **Reciprocity:** Another common tendency among people is the feeling that we should pay for what someone else has given us. Reciprocity is what is tapped into at those sample stalls at the supermarket; once you've accepted the bite of cookie or cheese tart, you then feel obligated to buy the product. If you don't, you'll probably feel distinctly uncomfortable saying thanks and walking away. This social norm of reciprocity is an incredibly powerful motivator and is used extensively in marketing everything from food and courses to raising money for charities and causes. The power of reciprocity is so strong in us that we can even end up buying things we don't want just to avoid guilt and social awkwardness.

➤ **Consistency:** Compliance professionals know that if they can get us to make an initial commitment, even a small one, we are likely to defend that decision – whether it was rational or irrational – to maintain consistency. Once we have taken an action or made a decision, we have a deep desire to appear to be consistent with whatever it is we have done. Basically, once we buy into an idea, we will often defend it all costs. We do this for a couple reasons. One, having decided on something means that we no longer have to put any more thought into it. This could take the form of brand loyalty or even an 'eating style'; we establish a habit, and that's it. Secondly, rethinking things can sometimes bring disturbing truths into the foreground, making it difficult to save face unless we change our position. In this way, we avoid thinking by acting out of habit.

Every aspect of consumer behavior is studied and analyzed by big corporations. How you think. What you buy. When you buy it. What your fears and pain points are. Is it your weight? Your health? Your desire to be a good parent and fear that you are failing? Your need for love and acceptance? Your stress level? Once analyzed, strategies are developed to increase the likelihood of your making a purchase, even for things you wouldn't normally buy.

We all have different triggers and different reasons for buying, and advertisers know this and how to promote their products in just the right way to make us say yes. They are very, very, very good at what they do, and they will go to great lengths to do it. It is safe to assume that nothing is random when it comes to product marketing and that this applies to every detail of everything you buy, including food. The colors, the text and the catch phrases splashed all over the packaging, the familiar faces (be they human celebrities or cartoon characters), the pictures of people just like you enjoying the product, the free gifts, the limited editions, the time and place at which advertisements reach you… these are all details that have been carefully thought out with your personal experience in mind – and their profit.

WE HAVE ALL BEEN MARKETED TO

Convincing us that we *need* things that we previously only wanted, triggering buying decisions and giving us psychological ways to explain our decisions, all the while making sure to maintain the illusion that we are free to make our own choices, is the epitome of successful marketing. Surely we're not that gullible, you say? Well, we are if we've ever eaten a breakfast of eggs and bacon, even very halal bacon. Enter Edward Bernays again, who was approached several decades ago by a company wanting to increase the demand for bacon. Bernays turned to the company's in-house doctor and asked if a heavier breakfast might be more beneficial for the public. The doctor approved his 'recommendation' and got a bunch of other doctors to do the same. The authoritative endorsement to eat 'bacon and eggs' was published in the media, and the rest is history! [22]

A similar campaign was run by the DeBeers Group, an international corporation that mines and sells diamonds. In the 1930s, diamonds were seen as an extravagance, and sales were at an all-time low, so the company needed a new marketing strategy. DeBeers hired an advertising agency to start a campaign. Through intensive research into social attitudes toward diamonds, the agency came up with the idea to link diamonds to love and paint them both as eternal. The catch phrase 'A Diamond is Forever' was born and is used to this day, making it one of the longest standing and most successful marketing campaigns in human history. Since then, every girl has had an uncanny desire for a diamond ring.[23] 'Because you're worth it'… 'It's finger lickin' good'… 'Just do it' – these slogans need no explanation. We have all been marketed to.

THE LITMUS TEST AND AWARENESS

Before we can take back our health, we need to take back our rationality! Ask yourself about foods you plan to buy, do I need this? Why do I want it? Where is this desire coming from? Is this desire rational, or have I been duped?

PAY ATTENTION

Pay attention to what you are allowing into your mind – ads, articles, television, social media. There is a reason why companies pay millions for a TV ad of only a few seconds at prime time. If it didn't work, you can rest assured, they would not be spending the money. Keep the principles of influence in mind, and be particularly wary when you find yourself being emotionally swept up in an idea. In this age of information overload, false news and deceptive marketing, we need to be extra vigilant about the influence mass media may have on us.

OVERWHELMED, TIRED AND COMPLIANT CONSUMERS

Of course, it's not easy to pay attention. Most of us are constantly running and feel overwhelmed. We have endless to-do lists and are constantly being bombarded by more: more to do, to think about, to see, to read, to try, to study, to eat, to buy. Businesses have a vested interest in keeping us busy and overwhelmed because, when we are distracted, running to keep up and just trying to get through the day in one piece, we are particularly susceptible to automatic triggers. Not surprisingly, when we are in this state and someone steps in with an offer to save us time, effort and energy, we are going to take it. When we are tired, we are also likely to reach for food that gives us an instant rush of energy and feeling of satisfaction – food that unfortunately tends to be primarily refined carbohydrates and unhealthy fat. The entire commercial industry has everything to gain by keeping us busy, strung out and wanting.

What the Food Industry Would Have Us Believe

"You're so busy, you don't have time, you have more important things to do than cook – but don't worry, we will cook for you!"

The industry tells us, "You have more important things to do than cook," and there is a social norm that spending time in the kitchen is degrading, menial and boring. The food industry has every reason to convince us that cooking is tiresome, boring and a waste of our time, or that it's just too hard. Once we believe that, we are primed to hear, "Don't worry, we're here to make your life easier. We'll do it for you!" Food is big business, and maintaining this rhetoric while offering to cook our food is the way a corporation can maintain its sales. Industrial help may seem convenient in the short term, but what they don't advertise is the fine print: "Eat now, pay later." So much of the commercially processed food they are selling us is slowly sapping our health, making us gain weight, affecting our mood and costing us more both in money and health in the long run. How can we stand up to this rhetoric? Rekindle the value of the beautiful act of cooking. After all, in the words of Michael Pollan, "Is there any practice less selfish, any labor less alienated, any time less wasted, than preparing something delicious and nourishing for people you love?" [24]

"It's so hard to be healthy. Healthy eating is complicated. You can't do it without us."

Even our health is being sold to us with the help of rhetoric. Nutrition advice with its complex portions, ratios, calculations, changing lists of what is and isn't healthy, and everyone telling us something different drives us to the point that we feel we need a diploma or degree to be able to navigate food and make healthy choices. I certainly felt that way… and I got that qualification! But the Prophet ﷺ did not agonize over nutrients.

Those eating traditional diets over the past thousands of years did not agonize over nutrients. Healthy eating is NOT complicated, and generally speaking, you do not need a nutrition expert to tell you how to avoid unhealthy food once you understand that the easiest (and simplest) way to avoid all that is unhealthy is merely to avoid the majority of highly processed, ready-made food and rather to choose whole food in its natural form. You may need some help re-skilling and learning how to source and cook natural food, and understanding portion control but, once you know that, you're good to go. The key to health lies in eating simple, natural food the way Allah made it, exactly as the Prophet ﷺ has advised us. And the foundation of healthy eating is not complicated at all. In the case of having already developed a health condition, this foundation of healthy eating remains the same, but there is also additional scope for therapeutic nutrition to support the healing process. When we are eating for recovery, support from a qualified nutrition consultant can be particularly beneficial.

There is a bigger change you make when you reform your eating habits; commercial producers don't profit from you when you buy or grow natural whole food. You're no longer buying their promise of good taste nor even their promise of good health. You're not even buying their wildly expensive, organic, ready-made superfood mixes. You're heading for the whole food section or going to your local farmers' market. You're buying from the source and cutting out the middle man. When you do that, you are no longer a compliant paying customer. Your natural simple diet means no more money for commercial food producers, and it also means that you'll gain health and energy, reducing your need for medication and denting a hole in another multi-billion-dollar industry, big pharma.

"It's your sedentary lifestyle."

There has been a move in recent years to try and deflect the blame of the health crisis away from food on to our sedentary lifestyle. While there is no doubt that we are moving a lot less than we used to, and less than we need to, simply put, you cannot exercise your way out of a bad diet. Many in the food industry would love us to believe that it's the sitting that will kill us – not so much the double-decker burger flanked by fries and cola.

We are easily influenced and often take information at face value, especially if it allows us to continue in our established habits. Take, for example, a flyer I saw in a fast food outlet announcing its encouragement of children being active. At surface value, this seems like a wonderful, socially-responsible thing to do, doesn't it? But, if we think about it, what does a fast food company care about our health while it sells food loaded with refined carbohydrates, unhealthy fat, excess sugar and salt and markets directly to kids? Does a company really care about our health that sells consumers a liter-size soda, containing up to 30 teaspoons of sugar, with a single meal?? Or, is it merely rhetoric to say, "It's not your diet but your lack of exercise that is causing your health problems, and we want to help you get healthy by encouraging you to exercise more. Now, would you like to upsize that meal?"

"You have to eat diet food to lose weight."

The diet food industry is booming, yet people are struggling with weight more than ever. Industries prey on our self-esteem and offer fabulous solutions in every shape, form and flavor, yet certain ingredients in diet food have been linked to weight gain, not loss.[25]

And there is so much more...

They Know Consumers Are Conscientious

Beyond all our irrationality, we are still capable of rationality. Producers know this and are wary of what might deter us from buying. They know we are compassionate and have ethics and that we wouldn't want to eat the chicken they are selling if we knew that the bird was bred to grow so quickly that it's body couldn't support its weight, lived a miserable life never seeing the light of day, had its beak clipped and had to be fed routine antibiotics to keep it 'healthy'. They know we don't want to eat lab-manipulated, genetically modified food that has not been tested for long-term safety.

They also know how to get around all that with clever marketing. When you select beautifully packed chicken breasts that read 'farm fresh' and show a photo of a chicken (beak intact) in a green farmyard with a homey-looking barn in the background, you have been duped. That picture reflects pure marketing as that's what we want to see. Yet, more than 95% of chickens are 'commercially farmed', which means the fryer or carton of eggs you're buying, unless organic and pasture raised, is not from a chicken who scratched about in a sunny field eating bugs with other happy chickens. A photo of the reality on the package, I suspect, would result in an almost 100% drop in sales.

Eat Now, Pay Later

Of course, not all marketing is bad. There are many ethical companies out there who are working hard to provide quality products and maintain ethical production practices. The problem is that the vast majority are not, and so much of what is being advertised is not only *not* nutritious and health promoting but actually harmful to our health – it's designed to look good, taste good, last longer and keep us coming back for more, at the lowest possible production cost to the industry. For example, the high fructose corn syrup in our drinks does not benefit us in any way. It's a cheap way to produce drinks that are highly addictive, calorie rich and very sweet and tasty even in the absence of any nutrients. It's a cheap way to make money. And not only do we *not* benefit, this 'food' harms us. Eat now, pay later. For a moment of sweetness, the ultimate cost is our energy, our vitality and inevitable decline in our health. We see the cost all around us as loved ones develop food-related illness and disease. We see the cost as children in our community are developing Type 2 Diabetes. We see the cost in the statistics that show cardiovascular disease and cancer are steadily increasing as we move further and further away from eating food the way Allah made it, the way the Prophet ﷺ ate it.

Remember that most corporations selling you food do not have your health in mind – their responsibility is to their shareholders and they must increase profits any way they can, even by producing cheap food that is not healthy and getting you to buy more of it, more often. They will delude via distraction, deception and false promises exactly in the style of the shaitan. And who but shaitan has more to gain from our increase in distraction and decrease in energy?

Our Part

We can't lay *all* the blame on corporations nor on shaitan. We have played our part, too, often knowing that we are not making healthy choices but choosing to make them anyway. We have an incredible capacity, when we want something, to switch off our mind to its potentially harmful consequences or to find creative ways to justify our decisions, a phenomenon well studied in social psychology and well known in our deen. Corporations merely tap into our established tendency to be mental slackers in the face of otherwise disturbing realities; we are easily convinced, so they give us what we *want* to see and believe. Seeing a happy chicken on the packaging allows us to convince ourselves of a happy reality, meaning we get what we want: a guilt-free omelet experience.

Making Conscious Decisions

There is not a lot of money to be made from consumers who buy based on need and who choose to eat natural whole food in its original form, cooking it at home. By processing food, branding it, and marketing it, food can be sold well above its cost price, making a whole lot of profit for those who sell it. We see this not only with processed food but even with 'healthy food'; food is big business and organic food is even bigger business. The organic and 'health' food industries are booming as consumers become more aware of food choices and producers know that we are willing to (and expect to) pay more for organic food. This success has been the envy of large commercial producers, who have reacted by branching out into the organic industry, buying up smaller companies but maintaining the small company branding.

We Have Everything To Gain

There was a time not so long ago when the only food-related thing we needed to focus on was how much we ate. Not purity, nutrients, deception, added potentially harmful chemicals. We are now at a point where, directly because of what we eat, our physical health, emotional health and spiritual health are at stake. We are physically, emotionally and spiritually unable to be the best version of ourselves. Worse, so many of us are trying hard to be healthy yet still getting sick and still low on energy. We are living in a time like no other, and these times require vigilance. The shaitan will trick people in any way he can. We have to be aware, alert and armed with knowledge to be able to see through the deception we face at every mealtime and in every shopping trip. Clever marketing may always be out to get us to buy more, but for manipulative marketing to be effective, we have to be *unaware* of the tactics being used and believe that we are fully in control of our choices. We can't avoid the consumer environment we live in, but we can be aware of the trickery and influence and become conscious customers rather that compliant consumers. We can also work actively to reduce the 'noise' and simplify so that we are able to see more clearly, able to better prioritize and able to align our choices with our ultimate purpose.

Chapter 2

A Vision
of Health and Hope

Change is in the air. Actually, it is not just in the air, it is steadily making its way to our shopping carts, homes and plates, driven by a growing awareness about our food, how it is produced and its effect on both ourselves and the environment.

Conscientious consumers and community members are opening their eyes, reading labels, speaking up, protesting food additives, and choosing to spend their money on more wholesome food. Social and other media are exposing corrupt food production and the damage being done to us and the environment, and governments and corporations are listening. The EU and France recently banned a set of pesticides known to destroy bee populations.[26] Other pesticides commonly used on food crops have been banned due to the risk they pose to human health. The fate of one of the most common pesticides still in use looks uncertain since a jury told Monsanto to pay hundreds of millions in damages because their pesticide was judged to have caused cancer in the plaintiff.[27] Due to consumer action, we are also seeing the first plastic-free supermarket zones in the

UK, BPA-free packaging, school districts embracing organic whole food school lunches over processed fare and countless other moves towards reducing the harm we are doing to ourselves and our planet.

Consumers are increasingly saying no to genetically modified food, excess sugar, and harmful fats, and more people are questioning the ethics of meat, dairy and egg production. Amazing innovations like biodegradable and even edible shopping bags are replacing plastic. Backyard organic farming is taking off as people realize that growing food is not only much easier than expected but also ensures quality and costs a lot less than many store-bought options. Farmers markets are popping up more frequently, and conscientious buyers are choosing to support 'the little guy', local farmers with whom they can personally connect and whom they trust. More families are deciding to cook at home rather than allowing corporations to cook for them. Even fast food options have been influenced by consumer demand to change production processes and menu offerings. In essence, more and more people are saying no to commercially processed products that are sapping them of energy and making them sick.

It has taken a lot for us to get to this point. Commercial producers have done a lot of damage to the environment and a lot of damage to us, which we have unknowingly allowed. As a global community, we have fallen very far before finally managing to catch any foothold. Muslim communities have been some of the hardest hit with our rates of obesity and diabetes among the highest in the world. Not only has food been causing chronic disease, it has affected every area of our lives. We are not able to live life to its fullest when we fill up on food that saps us of energy. We are unable to be the best version of ourselves – the best mom or dad, the best husband or wife, the best son or daughter, the best community member – when we are struggling to get through the day on 50% energy because the food we eat, meant to be our fuel, is instead draining us of strength. The food industry has done an effective job of deceptively promoting this type of food. We are at the crossroads of one of the most critical issues facing us in modern times. We have the choice to carry on the same path we've been on or to choose the road that leads us back to real health: the path of nourishing food that gives us the energy, vitality and ability to be the best version of ourselves, to worship Allah to the best of our ability.

Change is in the air. As Muslims, we need to take our place at the forefront of this movement. We have been given guidance and the keys to good health in the Quran and sunnah, but, like so many others, we have been affected by the deception of the food industry. Alhamdullilah, there is an awakening in our communities as awareness grows and more and more Muslims realize that the food they have been eating is making them sick and they want to turn back to eating the way the Prophet ﷺ ate. Most of us know we have gotten off track but we also know theoretically where the solution lies, and now it is just a matter of taking practical steps, one at a time. This is that moment in time. The choice is ours to make and, we have everything to gain. Though I cannot beam you into the future to know what healthy feels like, I am excited and grateful to share what I and others I have worked with are experiencing: energy levels rise, mood improves, brain fog lifts and we are able to think clearly and focus better, we feel lighter and more able to cope with our day, we are able to get up earlier and fajr prayer is not so challenging. We have become better versions of ourselves because our energy and vitality are being supported rather than sapped by the food we eat.

Just like a smoker might not be able to imagine how it feels not to smoke or know the extent to which the habit is sapping them of health and energy, anyone can experience the same with food habits. If you speak to a former smoker two weeks after quitting, you may well hear, "I can't believe how much energy I have! I can't believe I was operating with so little energy and had no idea. I can't believe how much better I feel." A similar dawning can happen to us when we change our diet and lifestyle. When we improve what we eat and how we live, we feel better. We gain energy. We gain health. Our mood improves. Our ability to serve others increases. Our ability to worship Allah increases.

WE HAVE AN AMAZING OPPORTUNITY

- to make changes and gain greater health, energy, and vitality, allowing us to be the best version of ourselves, for ourselves, for others and for Allah,

- to teach the children of the ummah about healthy choices so that they have a bright future and can share that information with generations to come,

- to seek Allah's pleasure and reward for elevating our food choices,

- to make changes that could transform the health of our planet.

Alhamdullilah, the amazing thing is that good health does not lie in complexity but in absolute simplicity. Allah is the One Who Provides for us and the Creator knows what the creation needs. I believe one simple principle makes up the foundation for food-related change and has the power to completely transform our health along with the health of the planet.

The Key to Healthy Eating

Eat natural whole food the way Allah made it, the way the Prophet ﷺ would have eaten it:

1. With mindfulness,

2. In small portions,

3. Without excessive frequency.

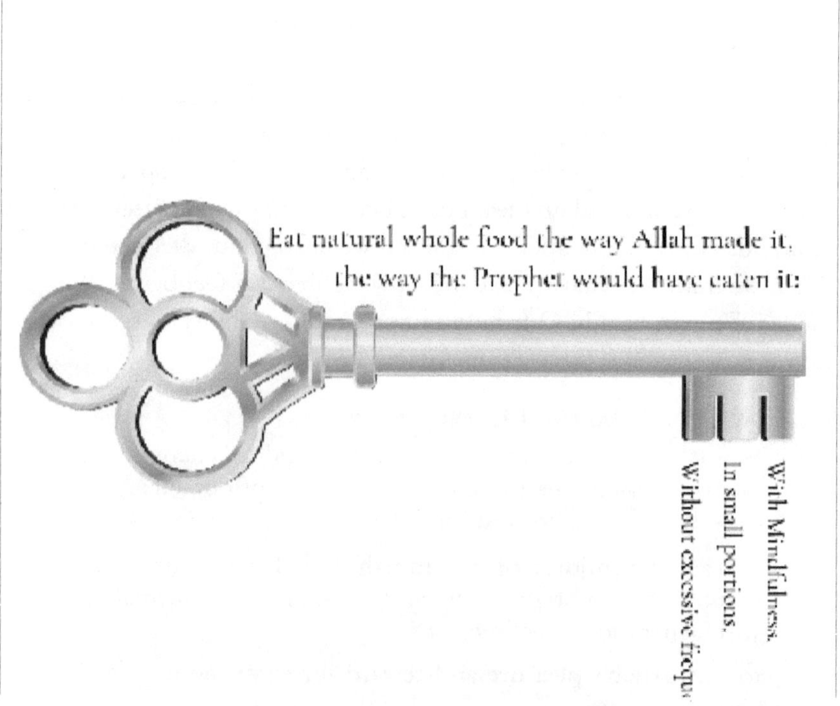

Allah has given us everything we need to sustain ourselves, and He has given us the very best example of mankind to follow for optimal day-to-day living. The Prophet's example of eating small portions and consuming meat only occasionally is indeed optimal. The key to good health simply lies in eating food the way Allah made it, the way the Prophet ﷺ ate, with conscious moderation.

Right now, the thought of making changes may feel daunting. You may be tired and struggling. Maybe you want to make changes and you know how important it is but you already feel so completely overwhelmed just trying to keep your nose above water. It may take all of your energy just to get up and get through the day with minimal achievement. Maybe finances are tight, you see no room for change, you lack support or just have no idea where to begin.

I understand how overwhelming life can be, so may I ask you to make a deal with me? *Breathe. Relax.* Read this book all the way to the end, but do not start making *any* changes until you have finished the entire book. No matter how tempting it may be to get started, promise me you will wait! It can be a bit of a bumpy ride finding out just how much is going on with our food system, but please trust me and stay with me on this journey to its end. Calm the inner critic and alarm bells if they go off!

Knowledge is the foundation of change, followed by intention, du'a, and action. To make long-lasting positive changes, we first need to understand the deceptive nature of the food industry, how we make choices, how to identify and avoid food that harms us and, finally, how to choose and access food that nourishes us. By the end of this book, you will have all of that and a solid foundation to launch yourself and your family into a life of greater health, wellness, energy, and vitality for the sake of Allah, one small and simple step at a time. Once you have the bigger picture in your sights, you will have the key to good health, the tools you need to make change and the mindset to ensure success, in shaa Allah.

Sister Khalida

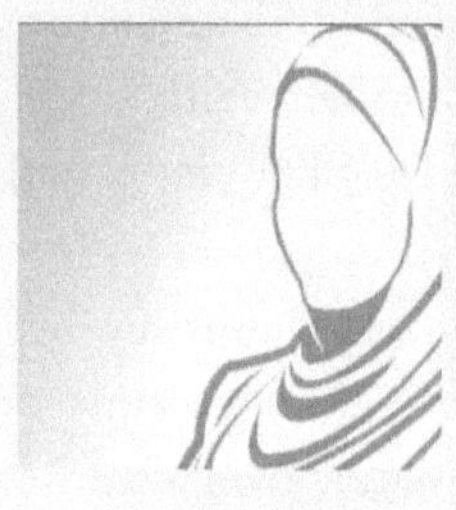

I am always 100% more successful when I do things one step at a time or in quantities that I can handle. I have spent an unknown amount of time feeling like a failure until I realized the problem was with my thinking. Two things dawned on me in the last year or so. One, small steps forward are still moving me in the direction I desire and will eventually lead to bigger steps. Two, I may not be able to read a book or start an exercise or eating plan and implement the advice given perfectly on day one. I may not even be able to adhere to all steps in the plan, but if I can follow 1, 2, … 5 of those steps out of 10 today, then maybe in several months or even a year later I can implement the rest. There is no rush!

We live in a society that tells us that it doesn't count if it isn't done a specific way or it doesn't count if the desired result isn't achieved in a specific time period. This is what I believe is messing us all up.

Chapter 3

Abundance and Excess

There is a fine line between abundance that begs our appreciation and abundance that reeks of excess. In our modern culture, navigating the abundance of food has become like walking on a razor's edge.

Allah has provided us with a plentiful supply of beautiful natural food that grows on our planet and, in all His Wisdom, has given every population of every climate and environment exactly what it needs. He has provided us with food that grows to produce not only food for the short term but also food for the future: each fruit, grain, tuber and bulb contains parts that we can plant to produce food in the next season, in an endless cycle of provision. Subhan Allah! Next time you eat an apple, think about the seeds you spit out. *Each* seed has the potential to be not just another apple but an entire apple tree, which over its lifetime may grow thousands of apples, each of which has seeds, each of which could be another apple tree. Think about that the next time you eat sweetcorn or watermelon or dates.

> *It is He who sends down rain from the sky; from it is drink and from it is foliage in which you pasture [animals]. He causes to grow for you thereby the crops, olives, palm trees, grapevines, and from all the fruits. Indeed in that is a sign for a people who give thought. (Quran 16:10–11)*

With industrialization and the commodification of food to the extreme, we have circumvented both seasonal and geographical natural availability to the point that everything is now available everywhere all year round. For many crops, to simplify and standardize production, producers have also chosen to move away from Allah's natural biodiversity and the immense variety that He has created, from thousands of varieties of grain, fruit and vegetables, to focus on monoculture: producing large, consistent quantities of the same few crops for the sake of 'feeding our planet'. Beyond the abundance of naturally grown food, there is an additional abundance of cheap, commercially produced food, loaded with added fat, added sugar and added salt.

We want it all and We Want It Now

As consumers in developed countries, we have come to expect that both commercially processed food and fresh food will be perpetually available. We would grumble if we found our favorite brand of cookies or bread out of stock and mutter about how the store's standards were slipping. We expect to see mangoes, lemons, avocadoes and strawberries in the fresh food aisle all year round. Imagine our indignation if we go for our weekly shop and find no lettuce or bananas and no fresh milk or eggs. Most of us don't give a second thought to the fact that fruit and vegetables grow seasonally, that much of the food we are eating has traveled thousands of miles to get to us or that, to create the enormous amounts we are consuming, these foods have to be mass produced, which often means using less-than-ethical techniques. Of course, we learned in primary school that milk comes from farms and bread comes from flour, but we don't often think about where it really comes from or the journey it takes before ending up in our trolley. We just expect it to be there. Every time.

There are many blessings in having so much food available to us, alhamdullilah, but this has also brought challenges. For starters, because we no longer have seasonal and geographical scarcity to keep us in check, with everything available in abundance all year round, we can easily end up over-consuming food, even 'healthy' food. Also, when we have so much, it's easy to slip into the mistake of complacency, becoming so accustomed to immense provision that we no longer deeply appreciate it or thank Allah for what He has given us. We simply don't remember what it is like to go without. It is easy to feel entirely self-sufficient when we shop at supermarkets, forgetting that it is Allah, and Allah alone, who has provided for us through His Mercy by the miracle of His creation.

> *And have you seen that [seed] which you sow? Is it you who makes it grow, or are We the grower? If We willed, We could make it [dry] debris, and you would remain in wonder. (Quran 56:63-65)*

DISCONNECTED FROM OUR FOOD SUPPLY

In this new age of abundance and variety, we have completely lost touch with the source of our food and our connection to our planet. For most of us, stocking up on groceries means a weekly trip to the supermarket where we cruise the aisles with our trolley and pick and choose whatever is on our shopping list, selecting from the immense variety of brands that line the shelves all vying for our attention and beckoning us to buy them over others. As we stock up, we are constantly making choices from among dozens of options for each product; not just one option for coffee but dozens. Not just one type of breakfast cereal but dozens. Honey that hails from all over the world. Twenty brands of eggs. Ten flavors of fruit yoghurt with varying quantities of milk fat – full fat, low fat, zero fat – and even milk free. Milk, meat, bread, cheese, condiments. Even with a shopping list, picking our way through this glut of choice is a challenge. With our time and energy already whittled down, most of us don't give a second thought to where this food came from, how it came to be on shelf 3 in aisle 4. And this isn't limited to the central aisles of packaged food.

In the fresh produce section, polished fruit is piled high under just the perfect lighting to make it look beautiful and fresh, though it may well have been in storage or traveling for 3-4 weeks or longer before being displayed for sale. And many of these items have indeed traveled far: mangoes from Thailand, avocados from Kenya, carrots from Australia, blueberries from the United States. Everything is available all year round – if we are willing to pay. Wintertime in northern latitudes is summertime down under; the dry season in parts of the tropics coincides with monsoon season elsewhere. Greenhouses anywhere use electricity to mimic any climate they want. Constant demand cannot be patient with limited growing seasons.

Nor does modern demand have any patience for naturally limited quantities. There is no better example of this than meat. When we order a bucket of buffalo wings, do we stop and think how many chickens had to be slaughtered to make our tasty starter? Do we think about the fact that our neatly vacuum sealed pack of eight chicken breasts is the result of four live slaughters? We may well be using several packs of chicken breasts each week on top of beef, lamb, fish and other animal products. In a non-commercialized environment, none of us would likely slaughter 4 or 8 or more chickens every week just to feed our families curry, stir-fry and burgers. But, because we buy meat ready-cut and vacuum-sealed, it's easy to completely forget that this food came from an animal (or many!) that was once living and breathing. This disconnection resulting from convenience packaging makes it very easy for us to overconsume meat, not only in grams but in lives, with many people eating meat daily and even multiple times a day, unlike the Prophet ﷺ, who ate meat only occasionally.

From fresh produce to commercially produced food and items imported from every corner of the globe, we have a lot of choices to make – and that's only our food. The sheer amount of choice we are faced with in every single aspect of our lives is overwhelming.

So Much Choice Isn't Making Us Happy

You'd think that 'more' would make us happier, but it doesn't. A child in Africa who can choose between playing with a stick or with an old tire is likely to be found smiling and laughing while a child in the West surrounded by books and toys is likely to be found bored and discontent. Similarly, those who live in poor countries and eat the same simple food every single day are often satisfied with their portion and grateful for their provision, while we have so much and yet we aren't happy, our food options having become a serious source of stress. While the poor feel satisfied with simple food, we may feel bored having chicken two days in a row, having leftovers for dinner or having no dessert. You don't see hungry children in third world countries complaining about dinner. They eat whatever is available with gratitude.

This phenomenon of discontent is explained by researcher Barry Schwartz in his book *The Paradox of Choice: Why More Is Less*.[28] He explains how the ever-increasing overabundance of choice we face in our modern world is turning our decision-making more and more complex and why so much choice is actually harmful to our emotional and psychological well-being, fostering feelings of self-blame and deep dissatisfaction that can result in mental paralysis and depression.

It would be difficult enough if all our available options were *good* options, but instead we face additional confusion over what is and isn't healthful and natural due to deception by the food industry. It's not a wonder we feel so overwhelmed with our options; it's like being blindfolded in a minefield.

Effortless Food at Our Fingertips

We have come to expect the store to not only be fully stocked but stocked with abundant variety, and we have also become accustomed to having ready-made food at our fingertips. We don't even need to cook our own food anymore, let alone grow and harvest or even wash and cut or sift. Anything and everything we could ever want to eat is available ready-made at the supermarket or cooked for us at the touch of our phone screen and delivered directly to our door within 30 minutes. This 'always available' phenomenon has obliterated the natural obstacle we would have had to overcome to consume anything in excess: effort. We can buy and eat anything we want without having to put in any effort other than swallowing... and perhaps chewing. But the physical effort we save with convenience foods we pay for eventually: either by the mental effort required to control our appetites or in the undervalued currency of our health and vitality.

Excess Everything

The commercialized environment we are living in has led to excess. In circumventing natural scarcity, establishing consumer expectations of year-round availability, disconnecting consumers mentally from the supply line so the reference point of 'normal and natural' is lost, making unnecessary the effort of preparing food and ensuring, literally, that we have anything and everything we could ever want to eat at our fingertips, with visual reminders everywhere we turn, we have been completely set up to overconsume, and that is exactly what is happening. It's not about what we need any more – it's about what we are made to want. Our choices are no longer about functionality or simple nutritious sustenance but about desire and convenience.

It's an ingenious way to increase sales: establish a global base of customers who expect everything to be available whenever they want it, then tempt them with unnaturally delicious food and assure them they don't have to work for it; they don't have to lift a finger except to click 'pay'. Who would say no that? Abundance is surely a blessing, and for food to be available in places where it was preciously scarce, we praise Allah and thank Him for food that helps us gain good health. Yet, modern-day 'abundance' has overwhelmed much of our capacity to be grateful; as consumers, we perpetuate the new status quo by virtue of our *expectations*. Expectations of abundance have resulted in excess on a global scale. Excess production. Excess consumption. Excess waste.

EXCESS LEADS TO WASTE

To keep our pantries and fruit stands packed to the brim just the way we like them, producers are producing too much, consumers are buying too much and, even with so much overeating, a mind-boggling amount of food is going to waste.

> *O children of Adam, take your adornment at every masjid, and eat and drink, but be not excessive. Indeed, He likes not those who commit excess. (Quran 7:31)*

Wastage occurs at every point along the production line. To keep afloat, farmers must do what they can to produce food that looks 'just right' because, with customers' expectations in mind, buyers are only interested in what meets the stringent aesthetic standards of the food industry. Because we have grown accustomed to fruits and vegetables looking a certain way, we don't want any knobbly carrots or bobbled tomatoes; anything that doesn't fit the mold gets chucked. Look at the carrots in your local grocery store next time you shop – chances are, you could probably use them as a ruler. Organic vegetables, on the other hand, tend to be anything but 'picture perfect'. The beauty of natural food is not in its aesthetic quality but in its nutritious quality – which, incidentally, tastes a lot better!

We can tut and shake our heads at producers wasting food, but in truth, we also have to look a little closer to home. We are likely all guilty of buying so much at a time so that we end up throwing food away. Be it moldy fruit and vegetables that we just didn't quite get around to eating or leftovers, quite a lot of our food can end up in the bin completely unintentionally. On a home-scale, wastage may seem innocent. But it adds up. In a 2012 report, it was estimated that 40% of the food produced in the US is thrown away.[29] Even more unsettling is a recent study based in Malaysia, a predominantly Muslim country, which showed that food made up 55%of solid waste disposed at landfills and that Malaysians generate about 15,000 tonnes (about 16,000 US tons) of food waste every day, enough to feed 12 million people 3 times a day.[30]

Sadly, the very worst time of the year for food wastage amongst Muslims is the month when we should be even more diligent. Ramadan has become a month of feasting, with iftar buffets popping up like mushrooms, homes kicking into full-swing food production, enormous amounts of food being eaten and yet enormous amounts still being thrown away. This can only happen when we have more than we need, when abundance has become excess.

Chapter 4

Just One Third

The Messenger of Allah ﷺ said: "A human being fills no worse vessel than his stomach. It is sufficient for a human being to eat a few mouthfuls to keep his spine straight. But if he must (fill it), then one-third of food, one third for drink and one third for air." (Sunan Ibn Majah) [31]

If we look back to the time of the Prophet ﷺ, we know that food was scarce for the Prophet ﷺ, his family and his companions. This is what Allah chose for them in all His Wisdom. We also know that the Prophet ﷺ is the best example of all mankind and those who followed him are the best of the people and that their level of worship was incredibly high compared to our modern times. What we see around us now is that food is abundant, most people are overeating, and levels of faith and practice of Islam are declining. If you wonder whether this has anything to do, even in part, with the food we are eating and how much we are eating, think about the effect too much food has on your worship during Ramadan.

We have all done it: tucked into an iftar buffet, eaten too much and then struggled to get through evening prayers. We feel heavy, we feel tired, it's hard to concentrate. Too much food eaten makes us sluggish, and it distresses our digestive system. It also inevitably leads to weight gain and the many issues associated with that.

IBN AL QAYYIM'S EXPLANATION OF OVEREATING[32]

"Physical ailments attack and harm the body and alter its normal functions, because of an excess amount of a substance. This type constitutes the majority of diseases and occurs because of overeating or consuming more than the body needs, that which brings about little benefit or is not digested easily, or due to complex meals, when the son of Adam habitually fills his stomach with these types of food, he will end up with various types of illnesses which take a long time to remedy. On the other hand, when one consumes moderate amounts of food and eats sensibly, the body will get the maximum benefit from this diet, as opposed to when one overeats...

The food we eat is for necessity, sufficiency or excessiveness. The Prophet told us that one only needs a few bites to sustain him, so that his strength does not fail him. When one wishes to exceed what is barely enough, he should reserve a third of his stomach for his food, a third for the water or a drink and the last third for breathing. This is the best method of eating both for the body and the heart. When the stomach is full, there will not be enough space for drinking. When one consumes something to drink on a full stomach, one's breathing will become difficult thus bringing about laziness and fatigue. One will feel heavy, as if carrying a load in his stomach. Consequently, one will be lazy in fulfilling his obligations and will seek other desires now that his stomach is full...

Eating until one is full harms the body and the heart, when it becomes a habit. There is no harm if one occasionally eats until one is full."

WHY IS 'JUST ONE THIRD' SO HARD?

We all know the 'one-third' hadith. We are reminded of it every Ramadan and find it among the classics that feature in every Islamic health blog. We all know it even backwards, and we also know that the Messenger of

Allah ﷺ is the best example and that everything he taught us is for our benefit. It's no secret that overeating is harmful to our health and is linked to weight gain, fatigue, gut health issues, obesity, diabetes, cardiovascular disease and so much more. So why, then, do we find ourselves loading up our plates at iftar buffets, having that second serving of biryani and squeezing in dessert even when we are already stuffed? Why do we find ourselves going back for seconds even though we aren't hungry, or scoffing a whole pizza or giant bag of chips only to regret it afterward? Why do we guzzle cookies and cake when we feel flat and reach for chocolate when we're upset? Even when we tell ourselves we don't want to overeat, often we still do, and we don't know why we are doing it. It's like we are on autopilot or something else is driving our decisions.

This behavior is, in fact, not random or inexplicable; there are clear reasons why we are struggling to eat less. If we want to try to follow this sunnah successfully, we first need to arm ourselves with the understanding of why we are eating more.

We Don't Know What One Third Is.

If we don't know what one third is, how do we know how much is too much?

The stomach is about 12 inch (30.5 cm) long and is 6 inch (15.2 cm) wide at its widest point. Its capacity is about 1 qt (0.94 liters) in the adult. It is capable of gross alterations in size and shape, depending on the position of the body and the amount of food inside.[33] Imagine a stretchy clear pouch with an almost 1 liter capacity, one-third full of food, one third water, and the remaining one third, empty space. If we take 1 liter as the relaxed non-stretched state of a human stomach, that would make one third around 330 ml (about 11 fluid ounces). The easiest visual reference we have of 330 ml is a standard size can of soda. This is likely a lot smaller than what most of us eat at each meal.

Of course, we don't know the exact measurement meant by this hadith, but the essence of the guidance is that a few mouthfuls are enough to keep our back straight and that, as a maximum, our food portions should be small. Using the size of a can of soda as a handy visual reference can be useful to help us consume less.

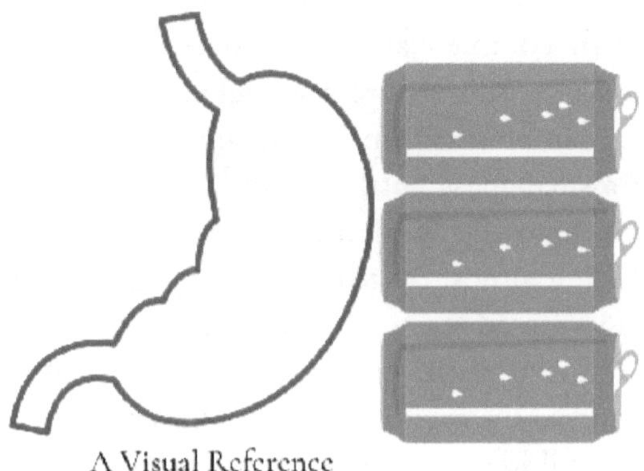

A Visual Reference

'One Third' is Relative.

Of course, the can of soda reference is not an absolute or a specification from the sunnah; it's merely a reference to be used as a guideline and a reminder to eat smaller portions. We cannot know with certainty the exact quantity meant by the hadith, but the essence of eating small portions is clear. It is also important to remember that how much you eat can depend on many factors including your age and your level of physical activity. A pregnant or breastfeeding mama or a growing teenage boy should need more calories than someone in their 50s with a sluggish metabolism. Those who are highly active will need more than those leading a less active life. When I did an 800 km walk in Spain in my early 20s, before I converted to Islam, I was eating an entire full-sized baguette almost every day plus cheese, pasta, protein and veggies. I ate more than I had ever eaten in my life. Yet, by the end of that walk, I was slim and muscular and very fit. My body had needed that level of consumption because I was burning energy furiously. Of course, I couldn't continue eating that amount of food once I stopped walking! I didn't need the calories, and I'd have blown up like a beach ball in the space of weeks.

So, how much food constitutes your *personal* one third at any given moment in time is relative and will vary according to the number of calories you regularly burn and also the nutrient and calorie density of the food you are eating. One third in lettuce is not the same as one third in meat, rice and other vegetables.

WE FACE PORTION DISTORTION.

Not knowing what a healthy portion size is has been seriously compounded by commercial portion sizes steadily increasing over the last 70 or so years. Burgers are way bigger now than they were even in the 50s. Fries can be small, medium, large or supersize, and we can no longer order a small glass bottle of soda. Some fast food outlets offer up to a liter-sized cup with a meal meant for one person – a full liter of empty calories including almost 30 teaspoons of sugar in one go. Because we are continually offered more, we tend to eat more, and when we become accustomed to eating more, we tend to serve more. When we serve more, we eat more and so the cycle continues. This cycle starts from childhood. In one study, children were given a child's portion of a kids' favorite, Spaghetti Bolognese. They ate the portion and then carried on playing. At the next meal, the portion was doubled, and, astoundingly, the same children ate the entire portion in front of them. In many cultures, food equals love, and feeding children is a mom's way to show her care and love for her kids. This is a beautiful trait based in the naturally loving and nurturing instinct that mothers have, but it's important to be aware of not increasing portions beyond what children need, as this sets them up for a lifetime of overeating.

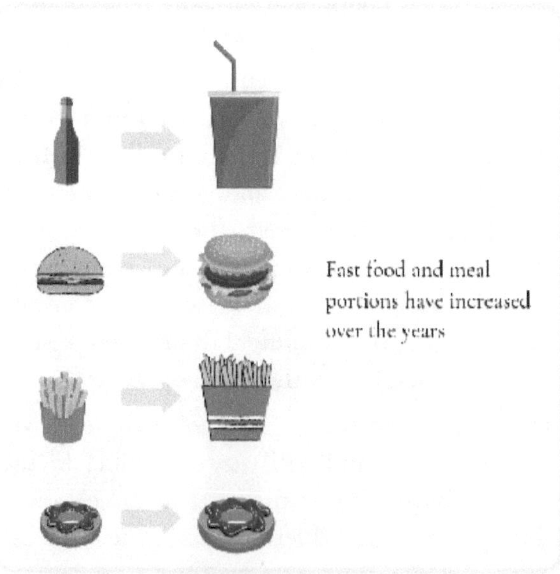

Fast food and meal portions have increased over the years

WE ARE ACCUSTOMED TO EATING UNTIL FULL.

Most of us have become accustomed to eating until full, so that only when we feel full do we feel satisfied. We tend to eat whatever portion size is in front of us, and because what's in front of us is generally too much, we typically overeat. This habit of overeating and eating until we are full starts in childhood and sets us up for a lifetime of overconsuming food.

WE ARE DUPED BY DESIGN.

Processed food is designed to be wanted, and wanted more. The food industry goes to great lengths to develop food that has been tweaked to profit-making perfection in a food lab, with just the right taste, texture and chemical properties to make us want to eat more and buy more. It's designed to be delicious and moreish, as anyone who's ever eaten a cheeseburger will know. Processed food takes advantage of our natural tendency to gravitate towards fat, sugar, and salt. Historically, in a natural environment, these ingredients would have been essential to us, enabling our survival and they would have been in limited supply because of natural scarcity. The catch we now face is that this fat, sugar, and salt are available in abundance, and they are heavily loaded into absolutely everything, along with tasty additives. The result is that we struggle to say no. Our struggle is the same as that of lab rats who, in one study, gained a load of weight when offered a 'cafeteria diet'. Instead of their basic, standardized laboratory chow, these rats were given chocolate chip cookies or other variations of energy-loaded, high-fat, yummy food, and, not surprisingly, they tucked in. Who wouldn't? The result was also not surprising. This simple change in their diet disrupted their normal body weight and body mass and triggered a 4-fold fat gain or more.[34] This is exactly what is happening to us as we eat, and overeat, processed food.

WE ARE NUTRITIONALLY HUNGRY.

The processed food that makes up a large percentage of most diets is calorie rich but nutrient poor, so while we may eat our fill, or more, in quantity and calories, often we are not getting the essential nutrients we need for optimal health. The result? Our body yells, "I need food!" and this translates to all sorts of cravings that we seek to fill. If we continue to choose low-nutrient food, we consume more and more empty calories but still miss the essential nutrients our body needs, and this becomes a never-ending cycle of eating and over-eating while remaining unsatisfied and craving food.

WE LIVE IN PERPETUAL ABUNDANCE

Not that long ago, there was natural scarcity because we lived in an agrarian society. Growing our own food meant we would eat what was seasonal and available either on our land or what was available in the marketplace. These days, the market has changed, and we are now surrounded by every type of food we can imagine in abundance all year round. Fresh fruit and vegetables – not to mention canned, frozen and dried – are available all year round, and we have come to expect this perpetual abundance. Food is available in shops and restaurants and by delivery and take away. Some restaurants and groceries are open 24 hours a day, seven days a week. While there is no doubt a blessing in having access to abundant food, this abundance is, at the same time, an immense test. If we are not mindful of what we eat, it can, and does, easily lead to excess. We no longer have the natural failsafe of seasonal scarcity to keep us in check, so we now have to be vigilant and use willpower to control how much we eat, even, or especially, when we are surrounded by always-available food.

WE ARE SURROUNDED BY FOOD.

They say 'out of sight, out of mind', but, these days, food is never out of sight and thus rarely out of mind. Images pop up on our phones, apps are ready and waiting to deliver whatever we fancy right to our front door in 30 minutes time, convenience stores overflow with snacks and ready-meals, and shopping aisles are packed to the hilt with anything and everything we could ever want to buy or imagine eating. There are food shows, food magazines, food courts, foodies. There's no getting away from it - food is absolutely everywhere. To make matters even more challenging for us, our digestive system is naturally stimulated by the sight, the smell and even the thought or discussion of food. Just reading about lasagna and cookies can start our stomachs grumbling. Those pizza ads with pictures of hot, gooey cheese are not random; they are designed to activate your digestive system and slyly motivate you to seek out the food you're seeing. With this constant barrage of food signals, it's hard NOT to have food on the brain, and when food is on the brain, we tend to eat more.

We are Disconnected from Our Food.

Another reason we often overeat is that we are no longer connected to our food sources. Because of commercial mass production and abundance, we have no reference point for what constitutes a healthy or natural portion. Let's imagine moving to a rural environment, or going back in time before supermarkets. Perhaps you would have a nut tree growing somewhere near you. The nuts would spend a season growing then fall from the tree, and you would have to gather them and crack open each nut, one by one. Only then could you eat them. It would also be likely that other people in your family or community would also be after those nuts, so you'd be sharing the resource with others. Think of this process versus buying a giant bag of almonds or pecans at the store and eating a cupful in one go, regularly.

The same would apply to honey, a blessed food that we love to eat, alhamdullilah. But think of honey in the wild. If, in your rural haven, you found a hive, you would have to smoke out the bees, and, after a lot of effort, you would get a piece of the honey comb, and it would be incredibly precious. Compare that to the never-ending supply we have available in the store. It hardly seems precious as we select a large jar from among dozens on the shelf and then dump three dollops on our morning porridge. Nutritionally speaking, however, a single portion of honey is only one teaspoon.

Now, think about meat. The Prophet ﷺ didn't eat meat regularly and certainly not daily or even multiple times a day like many of us do. Think about that pack of chicken breasts you used to make a curry or stir-fry last week. Let's say the pack contained eight breasts, every two breasts representing one chicken. Now imagine you lived on a farm. Do you think you would slaughter 4 chickens in a day to get those chicken breasts? Multiple times a week? Because we are disconnected from our food supply and generally don't give a second thought to where the food we are buying and eating comes from, and mass production means that everything is available in abundance, we tend to overconsume food without even realizing it.

WE EAT TOO QUICKLY.

We all know that it takes the brain time to catch up with the stomach and realize we are full, and we've all experienced that feeling of increasing fullness after a heavy meal to the point that we feel we are going to pop. What can happen when we eat too quickly is that we pack in way more than we need before our brain can say STOP! A good friend of mine at university had the philosophy, 'If it tastes good, eat as quickly as you can and get as much in before your brain can catch up.' This is an understandable philosophy for a student who's been living off of 2-minute noodles for months and only occasionally has the opportunity for a home cooked meal from mom. I suspect many have that same philosophy at iftar buffets.

WE ARE EATING FOR QUICK ENERGY...ON THE RUN.

Have you ever had one of those busy days (Maybe that's every day for you!) when you don't get around to eating breakfast, perhaps even skip lunch because you're running around so much and end up absolutely STARVING? When you get to that point, you'll eat anything! Once we turn ravenous, unless we are well prepared, have healthy food at hand and are conscious of our portion sizes, most of us are likely to make bad decisions, grabbing whatever is quick and easy that's going to give us the energy boost we need to keep going. Eating for emergency energy usually means we consume highly refined carbs, fat and sugar. Because we are so hungry, we also tend to eat too quickly and end up overeating.

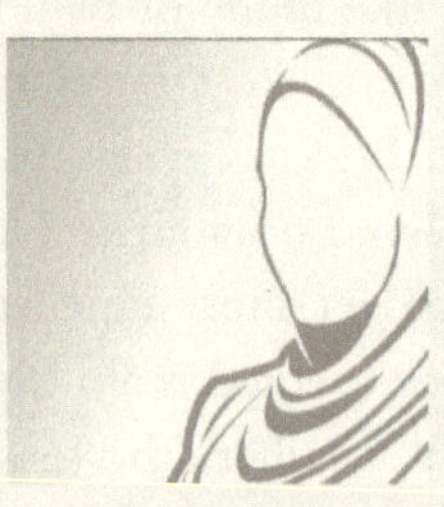

Sister Aaliya

Reflecting on how I eat, I realised how I don't really eat mindfully. It's pretty much on the go even if I'm sat eating - I'm thinking about something else!

WE EAT EMOTIONALLY.

For most of us, food is naturally attached to emotions. We connect food with happy memories, nurturing moments, social connection and celebrations. We all have family favorites and a love for certain dishes. Sometimes though, our emotional attachment to food can shift from healthy associations with memories to pure comfort eating when we are stressed, angry, sad or bored. Food can become a means of numbing pain, a distraction and a band-aid for emotional wounds that have not healed. When we are emotionally hurting and associate food with comfort, there is a powerful subconscious drive to eat to 'feel better'. This drive leads us to reach for comfort food. Naturally, this can contribute to over-eating and can make changing eating habits particularly challenging. Finding healthy emotional outlets and resolving emotional wounds are critical to establishing a healthy relationship with food.

Um Raqeeb

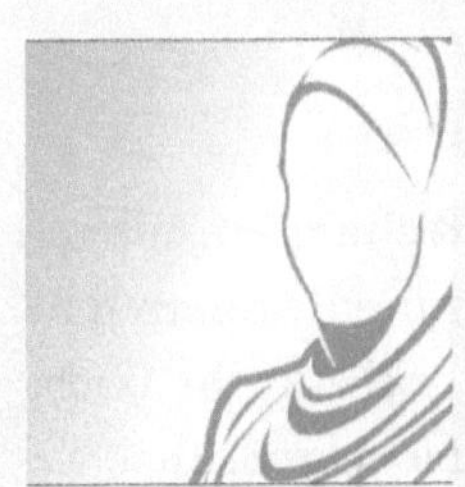

I remember that when I was small and upset or hurt my family members would hold me, hug me and always offer me a foodie treat to alleviate my distress. I now realize that very often it was their quest to alleviate their own distress because my crying was upsetting to them. Stopping my crying helped them and inadvertently they created a relationship between food and my comfort needs. As I grew older I would find myself reaching for food whenever I was bored, lonely, upset or sad. If I had a bad day at school I would want 'comfort' food when I came home. I developed a real hankering for sweets. I would go with my friends to the shop and we would buy 10p sweet bags which came filled with all sorts of delights. One thing I had to face was that by gorging on unhealthy food and habits I was not treating myself well. It has been a slow but poignant journey learning to love myself. This was not all about food. This was based and rooted in my own emotional ruts, my beginnings as a child and patterns of thinking that had developed way before I was able to recognize them. Food and my love affair with it was simply a by-product of it all.

WE ARE ADDICTED.

Eating is pleasurable, and foods are connected, to varying extents, to our brain's pleasure center. Refined sugar, isolated from any complex starch or fiber that would balance it, is especially addictive, and it is loaded into almost all of the processed foods that surround us. The comparison of sugar addiction with drug addiction has been widely studied and reviewed. To investigate why some people have difficulty moderating their intake of tasty foods, such as sweet beverages, researchers created an animal study where rats are deprived of food for 12 hours and then are given a sugar solution and sugary food for 12 hours. The result was that they learned to guzzle the sugar solution, especially when it first became available and after just one month, on this intermittent-feeding schedule, the rats displayed a set of behaviors very similar to the effects of drug abuse including bingeing, opiate-like withdrawal characterized by anxiety and behavioral depression and cravings.[35] Wondering if you're addicted? How would you feel if I asked you to give up carrots for a week? Apples? Chicken? Not too much of a problem? Ok, now how about sugar?

WE MAY SUFFER LEPTIN RESISTANCE.

Multiple hormones control how the brain manages feelings of hunger and fullness. One of these hormones, called leptin, commonly referred to as the "satiety hormone" which is produced by the fat cells in the body, "is supposed to tell the brain that we have enough fat stored, that we don't need to eat, and that we can burn calories at a normal rate." It also has many other functions related to fertility, immunity, brain function and others. As long as our body fat stays within a normal range, leptin functions normally and helps to ensure we do not starve. However, if we overeat to the point of obesity, the mechanism that is supposed to prevent us from overeating crashes. The body instead can become resistant to leptin. "When the brain doesn't receive the leptin signal, it erroneously thinks that the body is starving, even though it has more than enough energy stored. So basically, you genuinely feel hungry even when you are not." It also results in your brain decreasing your energy levels and "makes you burn fewer calories at rest in an effort to conserve energy." [36]

We Have Surrendered Control to Our Nafs.

In many cases, our nafs is in control of us rather than us being in control of our food choices and how much we eat. It stamps its feet and says 'I WANT.' Just like we train ourselves to control our nafs in the blessed month of Ramadan, abstaining from what is otherwise halal for part of each day, so too do we need to train ourselves when it comes to food and how much we eat. Like all training, this takes time, effort and willpower.

We Overeat to Avoid Waste...and Waste Our Health in the Process.

> *And eat and drink but waste not by extravagance; certainly, He (Allah) likes not AlMusrifoon (those who waste by extravagance). (Quran 7:31)*

Allah makes it quite clear in the Quran that wastefulness, a form of extravagance, is not pleasing to Him, even in the case that we are consuming halal food and drink or serving it to others. We are largely aware of that and hate good food go to waste whether at home or at restaurants, especially at iftar buffets! Mothers often pick up the well-intended habit of finishing their children's food to avoid waste, and brothers and sisters alike may be further encouraged to "finish the pot" by a certain hadith in which the Prophet ﷺ is said to have encouraged us to eat the remaining contents of a cooking or serving vessel so as to avoid waste.[37] But the Prophet ﷺ did not override his habit of moderation in the face of leftovers; we can expect he was referring to scraping a last bite of food from the bottom of a bowl, just as he habitually licked the last remnants of food from his fingers after finishing his portion, saying, "You do not know in which part of your food the blessing lies."[38] He was eager for blessings but not for a bellyache.

When we prepare more food than we can eat, we are faced, by our own doing, with a double-edged sword: displease Allah by overeating, or displease Allah by wasting. Remaining wary of portion sizes when purchasing, preparing and serving food and drink can eliminate the serious burden of wastage and help us to avoid overeating.

We Don't Realize Less is More.

Reducing food portions and increasing the nutrient quality of those portions is one of the critical foundations of good health. To do this, we have to know *why* we are eating more and take actionable steps to increase our success in reducing our food portions.

Not only does eating less help us physically to feel lighter and less lethargic with less strain on our digestive system, it also makes choosing better quality food more achievable. Purchasing less food overall produces savings that we can put toward higher quality food that contains more nutrients and helps us avoid harmful chemicals. Purchasing and eating less commercial meat allows us to enjoy better health while reducing negative impact on livestock and the environment. We can 'vote' with our dollars by choosing *more* food of higher quality while buying *less* food overall. This shift will pinch commercial producers. As we increasingly say no to their cheap but high calorie, low nutrient options, the forces of supply and demand will come into play, and producers will be forced to rethink the food they are selling if they want to keep our business.

We Cut Quality and Density Along with Quantity.

I had a sister get in touch some time back asking me how much she should be eating. She was trying to reduce her portion size to follow the sunnah but was feeling faint and dizzy and was seeking advice. As I said to her, the idea is not to starve yourself to create physical weakness or harm. If you are feeling dizzy and faint, reduce portions more gradually and choose food that is more nutrient-dense. A small bowl of lettuce does not have the same nutrient density as the same quantity of fish, rice, and vegetables.

We eat food to nourish and sustain our body. It gives us health, energy, and vitality so that we can worship Allah to the best of our ability. Overeating can harm us, and eating too little, especially too few nutrients, can harm us as well. This harm can be both physical and spiritual, so keep that in mind when you are serving up your food. The soda can guideline is useful to help us be aware of our portion sizes and not fill our plates — or our stomachs — to the brim.

Chapter 5

Then and Now: An Overview

Understanding just how the modern food industry operates and how it aims to influence our choices through clever marketing and social engineering, and knowing the reasons behind our overeating, are the two essential foundations to making positive changes. Next, we need to take a look at the huge extent to which food has changed since the time of the Prophet ﷺ so that we know how to navigate all the options out there and make the best choices we can.

Once we know what is going on with the food industry, we are in a powerful position to make changes, armed with knowledge, that will help us make better choices for the sake of Allah that increase our health, give us back our energy and reduce the risk of food-related illness.

It goes without saying that, in the time of the Prophet ﷺ, there was no need to differentiate between organic and commercially produced food, as all food was 'organic'. It is only with the advent of commercial food production that we have come to need the organic label to know what has been produced naturally and what hasn't. In the time that has passed since then, numerous changes have occurred, leaving modern-day foods similar to their predecessors merely in name.

Then	Now
Naturally processed food (like yogurt and bread)	Highly processed food
Unrefined food	Highly refined food
Natural food, natural additives if any (like salt, vinegar, spices)	Chemical additives common in commercial food: colors, flavors, flavor enhancers, preservatives, emulsifiers, food conditioners, mold inhibitors, etc.
Natural plants the way Allah made them, free from harmful chemicals	Chemical pesticides on plants and grain for animal feed
Natural food the way Allah made it	Genetic modification of food crops
Natural variety and biodiversity	Monoculture
Higher nutrient content of food	Fewer nutrients in natural food
No refined sugars or excess, physical scarcity of sweet food	Excess refined sugars common in commercial processed food and drinks (refined cane and beet sugar, high fructose corn syrup)
Natural sweeteners	Synthetic sweeteners
Natural wholegrains in balance, limited availability	Refined and GM grains commonly consumed in excess
Natural fats and oils like olive oil, butter, ghee yogurt, milk and animal meat	Excess vegetable oil, trans fats, 'fake' oils, damaged oils
Natural full fat, raw organic milk	Commercial pasteurized milk, low-fat dairy, hormones and antibiotics used in milk production
Pasture-raised meat and wild meat	Commercially-raised meat, animals raised in confinement and fed GM grains, treated with growth hormones and antibiotics
Pasture-raised chickens and egg-laying hens	Commercially produced eggs, battery hens
Wild, chemical free fish	Fish contaminated with environmental pollutants like plastics and heavy metals; Commercially farmed fish given antibiotics
Natural and chemical free water	Water often contaminated with pesticides, pharmaceutical drugs, with chlorine and fluoride often added to municipal water
Natural and organic packaging, natural cooking implements and utensils	Plastics and other chemicals in food storage implements and cooking utensils leech into food and environment

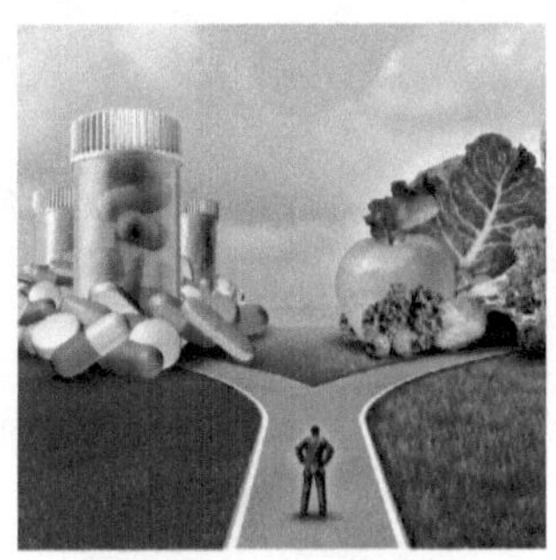

PART TWO
A CORRUPTED FOOD SUPPLY

Corruption has appeared throughout the land and sea by [reason of] what the hands of people have earned.
(Quran 40:31)

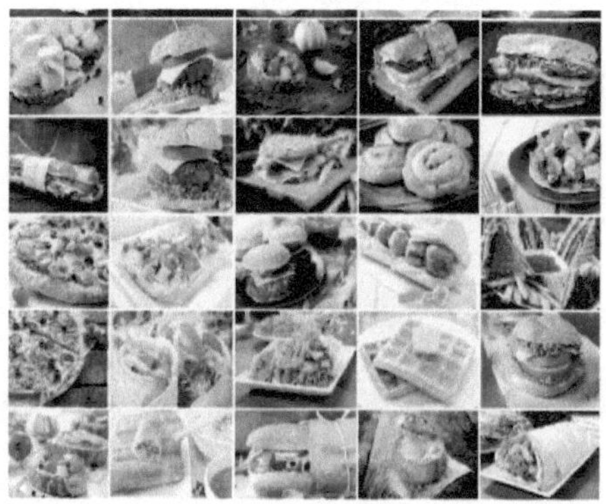

Chapter 6

Processed Food

Process/ˈprəʊsɛs/perform a series of mechanical or chemical operations on (something) in order to change or preserve it.[39]

It is worth taking a moment to differentiate between natural processed food and what we mean when we talk about commercially processed food. Any food that has essentially changed form has been processed: grinding wheat to make flour to make bread, turning olives into olive oil, fermenting cabbage to make sauerkraut, or allowing live cultures to turn milk into yoghurt. These and dozens of other methods of natural processing have been practiced for thousands of years. When we speak of avoiding commercially processed food, it is not this natural processing that we refer to; rather it is the modern industrial processing that includes refining grains, removing nutrients and manipulating end products with chemical cocktails and unnatural processes. Aside from its name, a highly processed cheese has very little in common with a naturally processed cheese.

Chapter 7

Additives

The food industry is fully geared up to produce food designed in a lab to look better, taste better and last longer. As consumers, we have come to expect variety, freshness, consistency of flavor and color and year-round availability for all the food we buy. Most of us probably don't think twice about how it is that every glass of orange juice from a particular brand tastes identical to the one we drank last week, last month and last year, even while we notice that flavor isn't always consistent from one orange we buy to another. How then do companies manage to create flavor-consistency from hundreds of thousands of pieces of fruit grown in different places at different times of the year? How is it that every sauce tastes exactly the same, every burger the same, every flavored yogurt the same?

The ability to deliver a wide variety of food sourced from all over the world that looks and tastes consistent, appeals to our taste buds, can be transported across the planet without going bad and is able to sit on shelves for months or even years without rotting is only possible because of additives.

These additives can do extraordinary things. They can make food last… and last, and last. I remember years ago, while living in London, I bought a loaf of super soft, snowy white sliced bread of the factory-made variety. That deliciously soft, fluffy, ready-sliced yumminess somehow got misplaced and ended up on the top shelf, way above my line of sight, and I forgot about it, only to discover it weeks later. On reaching for the bag, I imagined, in horror, an enclosed universe of mold. But to my worse horror, there wasn't even a speck! No colorful colonies. No crusty bits. No bad smell. Absolutely *nothing* about it would indicate that it had been hanging out on a shelf for weeks. It looked as fresh as the day I bought it. I remember thinking, what on earth do they put in this? I don't think I ever bought that brand again.

Starting to read labels was a pivotal point in my health journey. I took notice of the long lists of ingredients on packaged food, which included many words I couldn't pronounce or even identify as food, and I wondered, 'What is this? Why is it in my food? What is it doing to me?" The more I thought about it, the more perplexing the long lists of ingredients became. If you've ever made bread from scratch, you'll know that it contains 3 basic ingredients: water, flour and salt. If you've ever made a chocolate cake from scratch, you'll know the ingredients are flour, sugar, butter, eggs, milk, cocoa powder, vanilla, baking powder and a pinch of salt. Compare that to the list of ingredients on packages of factory-produced bread or ready-mix cake. If you have a loaf of bread or cake mix in your pantry, go check out the ingredient list!

ADDITIVES THEN AND NOW

It would not be accurate to say that additives are an entirely modern development. Natural additives have long-featured as part of a whole food diet with products such as salt and vinegar historically used to preserve food, along with non-additive preservation techniques like fermenting and smoking. These traditional additives and methods are still used to this day to naturally extend the shelf life of otherwise quick-to-spoil foods like vegetables, meat and dairy. Though cultures worldwide have used natural processes to preserve food for thousands of years, the vast majority of what was eaten in the past would have been fresh, seasonal and locally grown. The move away from an agrarian lifestyle to our modern age of industrialization, mass production and global trade has completely changed the landscape of food production and preservation.

The additives in our food today do a whole range of things beyond mere preservation. They enhance, flavor, emulsify, texturize and color what we eat. Although governments have banned many synthetic food additives that were used in the past, there are still a number suspected of being linked to poor health conditions.

Even food you don't think has addives has additives.

The bread loaf and cake mix in your pantry are only the tip of the iceberg. If additives have made it into our homes, we can expect they have also made their way into restaurants. Some restaurant foods, even fast foods may seem like 'safe' items that couldn't possibly contain additives. Take fries. Potatoes, oil and salt, right?

Well, here is the ingredient list for MacDonald's fries:

> Potatoes, Vegetable Oil (Canola Oil, Corn Oil, Soybean Oil, Hydrogenated Soybean Oil, Natural Beef Flavor [Wheat and Milk Derivatives]*), Dextrose, Sodium Acid Pyrophosphate (Maintain Color), Salt. *Natural beef flavor contains hydrolyzed wheat and hydrolyzed milk as starting ingredients.[40]

Flavors and Flavor Enhancers

Added flavors can be either natural or synthetic. Natural means that they are derived from nature rather than designed in a lab. So, we would expect the natural vanilla flavor to be derived from the vanilla plant that we find in nature. In actuality, it is sometimes derived from a very different but equally natural source: the gland near a beaver's anus. It goes without saying, when you buy anything 'vanilla-flavored', you probably aren't expecting to ingest beaver behind. The good news is that Castoreum, the official name of the extract is costly to produce and so not likely to be used in commercial food production.[41] Unfortunately, vanilla extract derived from real vanilla is also costly to produce, so we are essentially left wondering about the origins of any vanilla-flavored additive. While there may not be anything theoretically wrong with eating Castoreum, the mystery surrounding it does highlight that the word 'natural' technically covers a wider range of 'natural' than we might have imagined, and 'all natural' ingredients may not be the ingredients you would choose if you knew what they really were.

If flavors were not elusive enough, 'flavor enhancers' can leave anyone confused. One of the most controversial, and therefore familiar, flavor enhancers is MSG, monosodium glutamate. While some claim it is entirely safe for the body and brain, some people have exhibited sensitivity to it and suffered unwanted side effects.

Trying to avoid MSG and other additives was another turning point in my health journey. I have a deep love for taco spice, and it had long been a staple in my cooking. I had always bought ready-made taco spice, but once I decided to avoid additives, I could not find a single brand to buy. In desperation, I turned to Google wondering if I could try to make it myself. I was stunned to see dozens of taco spice recipes. I had no idea that such a magical taste contained just a few simple ingredients and took less than a minute to make. That moment transformed me. Not only did I realize that it was possible to make things from scratch but that it was also easy. I realized that I didn't need to rely on commercial producers to achieve the flavors I loved. I could make them myself, with higher quality and less cost and with surprising ease, alhamdulillah.

Sweeteners

High fructose corn syrup, other sugars and synthetic sweeteners are common additives in commercially produced food and are discussed in detail in the next section.

Colors

Like Allah's creations, today's commercially-processed foods represent the full spectrum of colors. Synthetic as well as 'natural' colors are typical. Rainbow-colored candies, pinked-up sausages and brightly colored sodas are all colored with additives with many artificial colours being linked to health issues in children and the wider public.[42] Colors are even added to fruit juices and other naturally colorful foods to ensure standardization. How comfortable would you feel as a consumer if the carbonara sauce you love varied in hue from jar to jar? Fresh food naturally varies in color, but we have become accustomed to uniformity, and color additives allow for visual consistency. They also improve the appearance of food and, in some cases, make visually palatable what we would otherwise not be inclined to eat, as anyone who has witnessed a hotdog production line will agree.

Colors are not only used in your food but *on* your food. Oranges are sometimes sprayed to make them, well, more orange, because we associate bright color with freshness, ripeness, and quality. Nobody wants to buy a pale orange even if it tastes like any other. Producers know that and simply aim to meet our expectations.

Historically, it has been the policy of the Food and Drug Administration to allow the artificial coloring of the skins of ripe oranges. It is a common practice in certain orange-growing regions in response to climatic or agricultural conditions that cause oranges to mature while still green in color. The coloring of the skins is done in one of two ways:

1. Adding a synthetic color called Citrus Red No. 2 (21 CFR 74.302(c)) directly to the skin of oranges. This is used if they are meant to be sold fresh and meet the maturity standards of the states in which they are grown.

2. Subjecting oranges to ethylene gas by a commercial process. This hastens the color ripening process takes place naturally after picking.[43]

PRESERVATIVES

Preservatives are additives used to prevent food from spoiling, growing mold, or decomposing. Commercial producers use a range of chemicals that keep your food looking, smelling and tasting fresh for longer than it would naturally. In the past, natural means of preservation, such as salt, vinegar and fermentation, were used, for instance to pickle a summer's harvest ahead of an otherwise food-scarce winter.

While preservatives have certainly allowed us to keep a broader range of food fresher for longer, these chemicals, particularly sulfites and nitrates, have raised suspicions. Sulfites can be of particular concern to asthmatics,[44] and the FDA has been petitioned to ban sulfite use in the past but they are still currently used in food. Adverse reactions to sulfites appear to occur mainly among a small percentage of asthmatics, but it is possible for individuals without asthma to be sulfite sensitive. There are also several other preservatives used in commercially produced food, many with questionable safety records.

NAVIGATING THE SEA OF ADDITIVES

Entire books have been written about additives, and numerous websites aim to help consumers navigate food labels, but, confusingly, there is never-ending debate and ever-new discovery about what is and isn't safe. In short, some additives may be safe while others are not. Diets that avoid additives and other specific foods have been incredibly effective in treating hyperactive and sensitive children, and, in general, additive-free, natural whole food is always recommended over processed food.

In his time, the Prophet ﷺ enjoyed less variety of food but encountered no labels nor any politicized confusion about what is and isn't safe. All food, even preserved food, was 100% natural, just as Allah made it, and subjected only to natural processes like ripening, acidification and fermentation. No potentially harmful or mysterious additives, just good, whole food.

One of the most stressful things I experienced when trying to shift to a more natural diet was the task of navigating and interpreting labels. Much of the stress we face when trying to choose health-promoting foods comes from the overwhelming confusion of trying to recognize, identify and judge the healthfulness of additives to processed foods. Not only is it stressful, but it takes an immense amount of time and energy from lifestyles in which time and energy are already in short supply. It is exhausting to read the label of every item you want to place in your cart.

Instead of navigating cryptic labels, I have found that I can mostly avoid them just by better navigating the supermarket itself. I have come to realize that roughly 95% of the food in the center aisles of any store most likely contains additives I would rather avoid; the easiest way to avoid them is to focus my shopping on the outer aisles. Fresh, natural whole food, i.e. food that is in its original form rather than commercially processed or altered, is more likely to be found at the outer edges of the grocery shop landscape: fresh fruits and vegetables, fresh meat and fish, fresh dairy products. Sticking to this plan most of the time and cooking with natural ingredients means you don't have to stress about long, complicated labels. It may initially take time to develop new skills in selecting worthwhile foods, sourcing new choices, and learning new cooking techniques, but it is entirely achievable if you take it step by step. It's certainly not as difficult as the food industry would have you believe! Improving your shopping habits does not mean that you will never buy packaged food again but that you will buy it less frequently and more selectively and, in doing so, minimize time and energy spent on studying labels. In the case of processed foods that you do want to keep on your shopping list, research the best options for you and your family. Look for whole natural ingredients on the label and slowly start building up a list of items that you feel comfortable buying for the sake of your health. Alhamdulillah, there are plenty of products that make our lives easier while also being nutritious and free from ingredients that we would rather avoid.

NAVIGATING ADDTIVES - STEPS TO TAKE YOU AND YOUR FAMILY FORWARD

1. Start reading the labels on foods you purchase.

2. Consider phasing out some of the processed food you eat and replacing it with whole food. Try out 1-2 whole food recipes each week.

3. Follow this general rule of thumb for additives: if a product is a psychedelic, unnatural color, contains a long list of unidentifiable ingredients, or features sugar in the first 3 ingredients listed, it's probably better to choose something else.

4. Start building up a 'safe' list of packaged items. For recipes you can't or don't want to make yourself, take the time to research the best options for you and your family. Look for whole natural ingredients on the label and slowly start building up a list of items that you feel comfortable buying and eating. It can be handy to connect with natural food lovers in your community and find out what they are buying. There's no need to go it alone, and gathering input from people who are ahead of you on the health road can save you loads of time and make your life a lot easier.

5. Become a label guru: if you really want to make sense of all the labels you encounter, there are entire books dedicated to understanding additives that you can dive into.

Chapter 8

Pesticides

If only labels told us everything we wanted to know about our food, then merely reading them should make food selection easier. Unfortunately, there is a constant battle between producers, governmental regulators and consumers regarding transparency. Consumers don't always win, meaning that we are sometimes left in the fog even when we've finally opened our eyes to these issues. When we eat fruit and vegetables, we don't expect to get a dose of pesticides with each bite. None of us would generally choose to eat food that we knew contained pesticides, yet many of us unknowingly do it every day, because food labels are not required to list pesticides as long as they are officially within 'safety levels' specified by food authorities. Even popular kids' cereals containing oats, as well as snack bars and 'healthy' granola can contain a significant dose of glyphosate according to an independent lab test commissioned by the Environmental Working Group (EWG) in 2018[45] and one of the main problems we face is that, while each individual pesticide may 'officially' be in the safe zone, the effect of eating multiple pesticide-containing foods and the risk of the accumulation and interaction of these chemical cocktails has not been established.

The worry of trying to navigate around pesticides in our food, and even having to think about them at all, is a modern challenge. Our great-great-grandparents, let alone our Prophet ﷺ, would not have given a second thought to the purity of the fruits and vegetables they bought in the marketplace nor worried that the grains livestock were eating contained harmful pesticide residue. They wouldn't have had to wonder if the food they were buying contained invisible chemicals that may be linked to cancer or infertility or that could harm unborn children's brains.

WHERE IT BEGAN AND OUR ROCKY SAFETY RECORD

Our history with pesticides speaks for itself. It's been a rocky road, with many chemicals once deemed safe and consequently used widely now banned or severely restricted because they have been proven to harm the environment and harm us. Amongst the most notorious of pesticides is DDT. Developed in the 1940s as the first 'modern synthetic insecticide', DDT was a massive hit at the time because it was highly effective in combatting insect-borne diseases like malaria as well as managing pesky insects in the production of both crops and livestock. DDT's glory was not to last, though. The superstar of 'modern pest control' fell from grace in 1972 when the Environmental Protection Agency (EPA) issued a cancellation order because the chemical was shown to be causing adverse effects on the environment and harm to human health. Following its ban, further studies uncovered a suspected link between DDT exposure and problems with human reproduction. Additionally, animal studies linked DDT to liver tumors, and as a result DDT is today classified as a 'probable human carcinogen' by US and international authorities. Unfortunately, this once-approved and widely-used chemical remains persistent in the environment, as it accumulates in fatty tissues, and is widespread, given its ability to travel long distances in the upper atmosphere.[46]

DDT is just one of several chemicals scientists have brewed up over the years that have come to be known as Persistent Organic Pollutants (POPs), aptly named because they have a nasty habit of hanging about in our soil, air, and water for long periods of time; persisting in the very foundations of our food system. Given DDT's grave side effects, its penchant for hanging about unwanted and its love of long-distance travel, it's not surprising that the use of the chemical has been severely restricted under the banner of a United Nations program to regulate

POPs. Unfortunately, the damage that has already been done cannot be undone. We can but hope to learn from our mistakes.

It's natural that producers don't want bugs, mice, or weeds overrunning their farms or fungi or microbes taking over. Neither do we as consumers. Unfortunately, the risk of infestation has actually been compounded by the practices of mass production and monoculture (planting huge fields of a single crop) as they unbalance the ecosystem, and monoculture is particularly vulnerable to being wiped out by pests. Allah's natural biodiversity, on the other hand, allows for a wide range of plants to grow symbiotically, and even if one is eaten up or harmed, it is likely the others will survive The 'solution' to these issues has been to use cheap, widely available synthetic chemicals, yet it appears they have ended up doing more harm than good.

Light at the End of the Tunnel

In all our cleverness creating chemicals to kill pests, we didn't think about the fact that they also kill birds, amphibians, fish and other animals, as well as bees.[47] Bees are of particular concern because they are essential to our food system. Allah honors these tiny creatures with a mention in the Quran, and an entire chapter has been named after them. In all His wisdom, Allah created bees as an essential element of food producing ecosystems. They do far more than produce amazing, healing honey; they pollinate plants, only after which those plants can produce our food. You see, killed bees means no pollination. No pollination means no food. No food means, well, you get the picture…we aren't going to last very long without bees.

There is light at the end of the tunnel as more and more harmful pesticides are being banned. In 2018, France's ban on five types of neonicotinoid pesticides came into effect, an effort to protect declining bee populations. The EU has also agreed to ban several of these pesticides, and this is a massive step in the right direction and a huge win for our environment, our health and our very survival.[48]

Also in 2018, the US Court of Appeals ordered the Environmental Protection Agency to ban the sale of chlorpyrifos, a pesticide commonly used on food crops.[49] Chlorpyrifos' safety has been the subject of long-standing debate, and studies have linked the chemical to brain anomalies in children[50] so this ban is excellent news.

It also looks like the clock is ticking for the darling of the GM food industry, glyphosate, a weed killer commonly used on food crops under the trade name Roundup GM. In a recent ground-breaking decision in 2018, a US court ruled in favor of Dewayne Lee Johnson, a terminally ill patient with non-Hodgkin's lymphoma. Johnson's lawyers had successfully argued that Roundup had caused his cancer, winning him $289 million in payments from the company Monsanto Bayer.[51] The most significant aspect of the ruling, and the reason for such a substantial order of payment, involves the claim that the company had been aware since 1983 of links between the chemical in their product and cancer.

RESEARCH CAN BE MISLEADING

Research is always done to test the safety of chemicals before they are used, so why did harmful chemicals ever enter the market, or, once put to use, why has it taken so long for some of these chemicals to be banned? Surely, when they were first tested, we should have known right away to avoid them? Unfortunately, it's not always that simple.

History shows that we sometimes get it wrong, and often it's only after a long period that we realize the extent of the harm done. For starters, much of the research done on pesticides is carried out by the companies producing them. Also, such studies generally test for toxicity in high doses over a short period, not low doses over a long period, as food-related exposure would more likely present itself. They also tend to focus only on the pesticide being studied without factoring in interaction with the many other pesticides we may ingest simultaneously, accumulation of those pesticides over time or their interaction with medications or any number of other environmental toxins. Studies furthermore tend to run tests on healthy populations. This short-term, single-focus approach to testing, based on a healthy sample, is not likely generalizable to the complex reality of our food environment, our exposure over time or vulnerable groups like children, the elderly, and those whose health is already compromised due to sensitivities or illness.

PESTICIDES IN THE TIME OF THE PROPHET ﷺ

In the time of the Prophet ﷺ, there were no synthetic chemical pesticides in use. All food was free of harmful pesticides. Now, billions of pounds of pesticides are used on food crops across the world[52] and billions of dollars are spent globally each year. The pesticide industry is big business with worldwide expenditures estimated to total more than $35.8 billion in 2006 and more than $39.4 billion in 2007.[53] These pesticides end up not only on our plates but also leeching into soil, running into rivers, affecting our water supply and the oceans and even polluting the air we breathe.

Without knowing the full extent of the environmental and human health impact of all pesticides, it's tricky for us to know what is and isn't genuinely safe. How can we possibly navigate these chemical cocktails when the science seems to be continually shifting under our feet? All we know with certainty is that many pesticides previously thought safe have since been banned, and more are being banned. But before they were banned, many of them likely featured on our plates, and many still do. At best, pesticides have a dubious safety record; at worst, they pose serious health risks and are vital contributors to both physical and environmental harm. While we have limited control over the environment around us and the air that we breathe, we do have choices when it comes to what we eat and drink and which chemicals we use in our homes and gardens. Without a doubt, the safest thing we can do is choose natural whole food that has not been sprayed with synthetic chemical pesticides, products from animals that have not been fed pesticide-sprayed grain and natural alternatives to synthetic chemicals for caring for our homes and gardens. By avoiding chemicals, we safeguard our families and ourselves, as well as the environment, from potential harm. By choosing food that is as Allah made it and eating it as the Prophet ﷺ ate it, we can't go wrong.

While the solution is fundamentally simple – eat natural whole pesticide-free food – achieving it can take a bit of time and involve challenges. It seems absurd that humans have constructed a world in which we have to actively seek out food that is not harmful and then pay more for it. Unfortunately, this is our reality. Making better choices is not always easy. When we are faced with opposing options, for example cheap commercially-produced strawberries (which we know contain pesticides) or prohibitively expensive organic strawberries, how can we feel good about our choice either way? Do we take a hit for our health or a hit for our budget? Or, do we scratch strawberries off our list altogether? We can only do our best to make sound choices given our budget and our living situation. Weigh up the pros and cons. Consider your budget, consider your options, ask yourself if this food is essential or if you can live without it. Explore any alternatives.

Quality Over Quantity

Purchasing fewer food products overall can leave space in the budget for pricier but higher quality items. Quality over quantity may be the best choice in the case of foods known to test high in pesticides, like on the 'dirty dozen' named by the Environmental Working Group. Strawberries earned the notorious first place on EWG's list of high-pesticide food in 2020. In the EWG study, one strawberry sample contained an unbelievable 22 pesticide residues and around a third of all conventional strawberry samples contained 10 or more pesticides.[54]

The Dirty Dozen List of 2020

> Strawberries, spinach, kale, nectarines, apples, grapes, peaches, cherries, pears, tomatoes, celery, potatoes and hot peppers

I would recommend trying to avoid items on this list as much as possible if you are not able to afford organic and, instead, spend your money on fruits and vegetables on the EWG's 'Clean Fifteen' list of items that tested with the least pesticide residue.

Clean Fifteen List of 2020

> Avocados, sweetcorn, pineapples, onions, papaya, sweet peas (frozen), eggplants, asparagus, cauliflower, cantaloupes, broccoli, mushrooms, cabbage, honeydew melon and kiwi.

NOTE: This study was done on produce in the United States so there is no guarantee that the same data will apply to produce in other countries. As such, for outside the US use it as a guide by all means but do try to see if any local agencies have done similar local studies.

ACTION POINTS

FRUIT AND VEGETABLES

- Grown your own. More and more people are starting up backyard gardens to ensure their food is safe and pesticide free. It's not as hard to grow food as you might imagine and is highly cost-effective.

- Connect with local farmers and head to your closest farmers' market. Fruits and vegetables at markets featuring local farmers are fresh, seasonal, and often a lot cheaper than store-bought produce. This is because organic certification is a costly business, so it may not be affordable for small farmers to get certified even though they adhere to organic standards.

- At supermarkets, buy organic if possible. Can't go 100% organic? Don't worry. Do what you can using the 'dirty dozen' and 'clean fifteen' lists as a guide to avoid the worst offenders. (For those in the US)

- Wash all non-organic fruit and vegetables thoroughly and peel if possible. This reduces the likelihood of ingesting pesticides.

- Avoid soft-skinned, non-organic fruit (like blueberries, raspberries and strawberries) that can't be washed thoroughly or peeled.

- Choose frozen organic produce over fresh non-organic especially for food with a high risk of pesticides.

GRAINS AND LEGUMES

- Try to avoid GM grains or GM grain by-products as they are generally heavily sprayed with pesticides. Choose organic grains and legumes where possible. Relatively speaking, organic grains and legumes are quite affordable and will not make a massive dent in your food budget, especially if you buy in bulk.

Meat

- Choose organic, pasture-raised animals where possible to avoid ingesting pesticide residue. Commercially raised animals are generally fed a diet high in GM grains which have been sprayed with pesticides, residues of which can remain in the meat.

Honey

- Choose organic, raw, unfiltered, unpasteurized honey, and head down to your local farmers' market or look up beekeepers in your area and connect with them directly.

Chapter 9

Genetically Modified Food

Farmers have long practiced traditional methods of plant 'breeding' such as combining particularly strong plants with others or mixing similar plants of the same species, to create a new hybrid. For example, tangelos are a hybrid of grapefruit and tangerines. The difference between these traditional methods and modern techniques is that scientists can now cross species boundaries that could not be crossed by conventional plant breeding. This means they can modify genes, transferring traits between entirely unrelated species, such as from bacteria or animals to plants. According to one definition, a genetically modified organism "is a plant, animal, microorganism or another organism whose genetic makeup has been modified in a laboratory using genetic engineering or transgenic technology. This creates combinations of plant, animal, bacterial and virus genes that do not occur in nature or through traditional crossbreeding methods." [55]

The most common commercial GM crops today are soy, corn, cotton, canola, alfalfa and sugar beets. These are largely used either as food for animals or as ingredients in processed food. If the label of a food containing these products, or their by-products, does not mention 'GMO-free', there's a good chance the ingredient is genetically modified. As with pesticides and other synthetic products, short-term studies resulted in a green light for food producers. No long-term safety studies have been done on humans, but animal studies suggest possible cause for concern.

Varied vs. Monoculture

Traditional farming methods made use of numerous varieties of the crops we know today and continue to do so in certain parts of the world, especially in Southern Asia. These 'heirloom' varieties have hardly been grown in the United States, however, since around WWI, as that is when industrial agriculture took off. Though small-scale farmers have made a decidedly reactionary effort to reintroduce some heirloom varieties of fruits and vegetables, a trip through a typical supermarket today will acquaint us with only one or two varieties of each type of produce, unlike the wide and very colorful abundance of Allah's creation – from pink, red and purple carrots to striped tomatoes and bananas in more shapes, sizes and even colors (including pink) than you can imagine. What is even more incredible about heirloom seeds and plants grown from them is that they also have different strengths – some are more heat tolerant, some resistant to the cold, some can survive in dryer conditions and all of these traits and genes can be used by plant breeders to create stronger (while still natural) plants that can survive and thrive, particularly important as the temperature of our planet and weather fluctuates from year to year.

Where there is biodiversity, with a variety of crops planted in neighboring plots, even if one plant type is harmed by drought, disease or infestation, other species are likely to survive. The greater the variety, the greater the food security.[56] With the ever-increasing drive to produce more with less, however, farmers have started focusing on monoculture, growing just one genetic variety of plant. This variety will be carefully selected based on its ability to tolerate industrial processes like mechanical picking and long-distance shipping as well as climatic and environmental threats. Monoculture is the reason we find only one or two types of banana at the supermarket. The risk of monoculture is that, in the face of an enemy, all the plants stand to suffer. By producing only one crop type, a single pest might threaten to wipe out the entire crop.

Resource for Heirloom Seeds: www.seedsavers.org

Monoculture Leads to GM Designer Crops

Using biotechnology, scientists have found a way around the risk of monoculture, by creating plants resistant to certain pesticides. The chemicals sprayed on these crops kill everything except the plant. Monsanto's Roundup Ready brand of GM seeds produce such plants, designed to be resilient to the company's Roundup brand weed killer. Technology has also allowed scientists to create plants that produce their own pesticide. For example, Bt corn has been genetically modified to produce an endotoxin highly effective at killing a certain caterpillar that likes to eat it, while generally not killing other insects.[57]

GM Farming is no doubt high-tech and is furthermore big business – designer business. It should not be surprising, then, that GM seeds are patented. A farmer growing a crop of GM corn is legally forbidden to save any of those seeds to plant the following year, as farmers have been doing for thousands of years. GM farmers are contractually obligated to buy a new batch of seeds each year.

GM Safety

While not all scientists agree that GM crops pose a threat, genetic modification of food is a relatively new technology, and, like many developments in food and agriculture, its safety has not been established on long-term human studies. The FDA classifies GM food as *'generally recognized as safe'* (GRAS), but we know they don't always get it right the first time. Though research results have varied widely, several animal studies indicate that GM food may alter gut bacteria, blood chemistry, organ weight, cause disturbances to the digestive system, changes to the pancreas and liver and kidney and liver toxicity.[58] Of course, we can't be sure that GM food will have the same effect on us. Perhaps we'll find out after a few generations! Other animal studies link the consumption of GMOs to an increase in allergies, ADHD, cancer, infertility, chronic immune disorders and more.[59]

GM Necessity?

GM products and their derivatives make up a lot of the processed food we buy today, though the majority of GM crops are not sold as human food but reach us indirectly. Around 70-90% of harvested GM crops are fed to animals.[60] Food producers argue that GM crops are necessary to feed the world, but in reality such grain is used to feed livestock to fulfill our First-World appetite for meat. Given that excess meat consumption has been linked to health issues, the single most dramatic shift we can make to reduce GM crop production is to reduce our meat consumption. By reducing demand, not only would the amount of GM crops diminish, the pesticides used on these crops would be reduced and the quality of livestock diet and lives could be increased.

GM SUICIDE?

Genetic modification has been taken to the extreme with technology such as 'terminator seeds'. Terminator seeds are named such because they contain 'suicide gene' technology. Instead of the seeds being fertile so that they can be planted again as part of the natural cycle of plant reproduction, terminator seeds 'commit suicide' after one growth season. The seeds they produce are entirely infertile, ending the natural plant cycle of growth, death and regrowth but ensuring seasonal seed purchases that would bring in profit and protect patents. It may sound like science fiction, but this technology already exists, and Monsanto owns the patent. Fortunately, the company has publicly promised not to use it in food crops.[61]

Assurances aside, it's not a wonder that the mere idea that such technology exists makes people nervous. It doesn't take too far a stretch of the imagination to think of the potential for disaster if such seeds were ever introduced to the environment. Bees and bugs would not know the difference and cross-pollination would be almost impossible to avoid. Could such technology result in an irreversible chain reaction of infertile plants, putting the entire planet's food supply at risk?

Genetic modification might have come about as the proposed solution to feeding the planet, but it has also come with a fair share of issues and areas of concern. In contrast to our biotech crops, food in the time of the Prophet ﷺ was 100% natural, just as Allah created it, and abundant biodiversity was the natural law of the land.

ALLAH MADE VARIETY

The high-tech, cross-species varieties made possible by genetic modification is not to be confused with Allah's infinitely wise creation of variety. For many of us, our experience with variety has been so severely limited by monoculture commercial farming that fruit or vegetables that look unfamiliar evoke feelings of concern and even disgust. Coming across an heirloom-variety yellow tomato with green stripes could be an emotional experience! As it turns out, there are actually thousands of varieties of heirloom tomatoes that are non-hybridized. Navigate Asian markets for the first time, and it's a wondrous experience filled with yellow watermelons, wildly purple dragon fruit and alien-like rambutans along with bundles of green leafy vegetables that nobody from the West would recognize at all. If, like me, you are a mango lover, you might want to move to India for a year – or four. That's how long it would take you to try out all of the 1500 or so varieties of mango there.[62] You could chew, scoop and suck different mangoes to your heart's content for four whole years, or at least as they come into season in different parts of the country.

We are so used to fruits and vegetables looking a certain way that when we see anything different, we may yell, "GM!" Little do we know that yellow watermelons, purple tomatoes and the 1500 varieties of mango in India are all part of Allah's amazing bounty. If you're looking for something to do, spend an afternoon browsing the internet googling varieties of various fruits and vegetables. You'll uncover thousands of wondrous variations of edible plants that you never knew existed and refresh your appreciation of the wonder of Allah's creation. Unlike terminator seeds, these natural plant varieties grow from 'heirloom seeds' which are genetically identical to their 'parents' so they can be planted again and again and again in a never-ending cycle of provision, alhamdulillah. Allah has created incredible natural biodiversity, abundance and balance.

KEY TAKEAWAYS

- GM is not the same as traditional hybridization.
- The most common commercial GM crops today are soy, corn, cotton, alfalfa, canola and sugar beets and these are either used as food for animals or as ingredients in processed food. These additives are not always easily identifiable.

- If a processed food does not say GMO-FREE, there is a good chance it contains GM ingredients.

- The long-term safety of GMOs is not yet known, but animal studies suggest there might be reason for concern.

- There is an immensely abundant variety of food out there that we have probably never even seen or heard about, and there's a good chance it's natural.

Chapter 10

Nutrient Density

While it's impossible to know the exact nutrient density of foods available in the time of the Prophet ﷺ, we can look at a more recent comparison for an idea of how nutrient content has changed over the years. As it turns out, fruit and vegetables are less nutritious now than they were even just 70 years ago.

A team of researchers from the University of Texas compared agricultural data from 1950 and 1999 for 43 different fruits and vegetables and found 'reliable declines' in calcium, vitamin B12, vitamin C, phosphorous, iron and protein since 1950. Evidence linked this reduction in nutrients to farmers' increased focus on factors like size, growth rate and resistance to pests, rather than to the products' nutritional value.

Efforts to breed new varieties of crops that provide greater yield, pest resistance, and climate adaptability have allowed crops to grow bigger and more rapidly, but their ability to manufacture or uptake nutrients has not kept pace with their rapid growth.[63]

The Organic Consumers Association cites several other studies with similar findings, and there may be additional causes for the confirmed lower nutritional content of today's food. There is also a significant difference in the nutrient quantity of organic and non-organic milk and between organic, grass fed or pasture raised animals and those raised on a high-grain diet in feedlots.

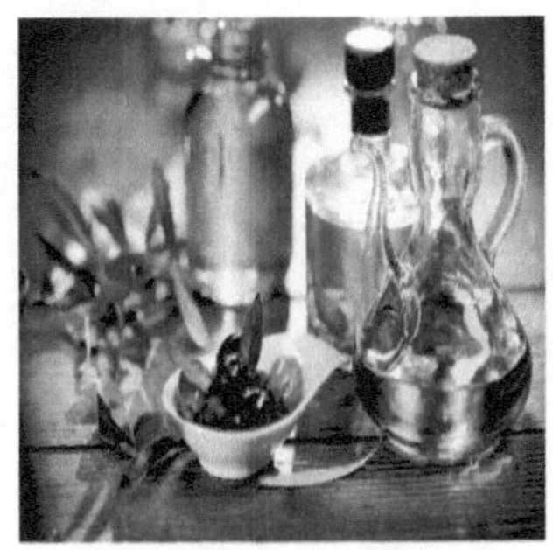

PART THREE
FOOD, THEN AND NOW

O mankind, eat from whatever is on earth [that is] lawful and good and do not follow the footsteps of Satan. Indeed, he is to you a clear enemy. (Quran 2:168)

In this section, let's take a walk through the spectrum of foods available today and consider how they compare to what was available at the time of the Prophet ﷺ. For each type of food, we'll discover action we can take towards improving our selection and preparation of food.

Chapter 11

Sugar

Sugar comes in two forms in our diets: naturally occurring sugars and added sugars. Naturally occurring, as the name suggests, are sugars found naturally in foods such as fructose in fruit and lactose in milk and others like honey, which contains a combination of fructose and glucose as well as water, pollen and beneficial minerals. Added sugars are refined or processed sugars that are added to food, sometimes even in addition to naturally occurring sugars, as in the case of chocolate or strawberry milk.

Sugar consumption has sky-rocketed in recent years. Looking back, in the early 1800s, an average person consumed just 10 pounds of sugar per year, and, stepping back even further in time, it's estimated that earlier ancestors ate only around 22 teaspoons of sugar a year. From 1815 to 1970, the amount of sugar consumed in England per capita rose from 15 pounds to 54.5 kg[64] and these statistics are similar in comparable countries. It's now estimated that the average American is eating 22 teaspoons of sugar *every single day*.

Where did everything change? How did we get to this point? Although the first evidence of production of a crystalline form of sugar can be dated as far back as about 500 BC in northern India, things didn't start getting out of control until the technology of the 1960s. New developments allowed manufacturers to cheaply mass produce High Fructose Corn Syrup, the incredibly sweet processed sugar that is now used extensively in commercially produced food from sodas to baked goods, canned fruits, jams, and even dairy products.[65]

This has had an unbelievable effect on our sugar intake. The consumption of HFCS alone increased more than 1000% between 1970 and 1990,[66] and it now makes up an estimated 40% of the caloric sweeteners added to food and drink worldwide. In the US, where HFCS is the primary caloric sweetener used in sodas and other soft drinks, the increase in HFSC mirrors the rise in obesity to the point that such high calorie drinks are suspected to have played a significant role in the rise of obesity.

You may be thinking this doesn't apply to you –you'd never eat 22 teaspoons of sugar a day! Well, you might be surprised. If you're eating a diet high in processed food, even processed savory food, you're likely ingesting plenty of sugar. It is added to almost everything, and it is particularly prevalent in kids' food, often well-hidden by clever packaging, deceptive labeling and ingredient manipulation.

TAKE A COMMON 'HEALTHY' BREAKFAST...

- Cereal: A single 30 g portion (recommended portion according to the label) can have 15 g of sugar in it (almost 4 tsp), but almost nobody eats 30 g of cereal. Most people would eat 60-80 g so, if we imagine we have a 60 g portion – double up and we have 8 tsp of sugar already.

- Add a small tub of low-fat fruit, and you could have another 15 g of sugar (almost 4 tsp).

- Add an 8 oz serving of orange juice, and you add an astounding 22 g of sugar (about 5 tsp).

For such a 'healthy' breakfast, you're already up to double digits in teaspoons of total sugar, and you haven't even made it out the front door.

This is a typical breakfast for many and a common 'healthy' breakfast for kids, but the reality is that this meal is sugar-loaded. On top of that, the grain in your morning cereal is likely a refined carbohydrate (the nutritious, high fiber bran layer having been discarded for the sake of texture), adding to the glycemic effect this food has on our body: the type of sugar in juice and refined grain, in the absence of high fiber bran and fruit pulp, rushes unobstructed to our bloodstream and gives us that well-known 'sugar rush'.

For many of us, that sugar rush gets us through the morning rush… only to leave us fallen and fatigued by the time we arrive at our day's work – and craving another rush. Take the sugar we had for breakfast, and add to that the sweets, cookies, coffee, tea and other food and drinks we eat during the day, and you can see how it's easy for any of us to clock up 22 teaspoons or even more. A single can of soda can contain 9 teaspoons of sugar, and many people, especially teenagers, are drinking multiple cans a day. Fast food outlets offer, with an upsized meal, up to a liter of soda which would hold almost 30 teaspoons of sugar in a 'single portion'. And that's just the sweet stuff. If you start reading your labels, you will see sugar in nearly all the savory food you are eating, too, hidden in places we wouldn't expect it like ketchup, mustard, salad dressing, and pasta sauces. It's even in foods that we may think of as 'healthy' foods. Low-fat fruit yogurt and granola and cereal bars are particularly deceptive, posing as health foods for kids while they are actually sugar-loaded, and even fruit juices, which are already high in natural sugar and missing any natural fiber to slow down the digestions and absorption process, often have even more sugar added to them in the form of HFCS or other sugary sweeteners.

Consumers are increasingly cottoning on to the added sugar and are starting to check labels, and so producers have gotten smarter. They have figured out a way to tweak labels to make their products look less unhealthy without changing anything about the product: Portion sizes on the label, on which nutrition content is based, are *small*, way smaller than anyone would eat. Producers know full well that you will eat more. They have also come up with a way to sneakily side-step printing 'added sugar' on the label. Instead, ingredients may contain 'fruit juice concentrate' with the selling-point 'NO ADDED SUGAR' splashed all over the packaging; yet fruit juice concentrate contains not just fructose but *concentrated* fructose and is adding to your daily load of sugar and affecting your body. There is an entire palette of sweet additives from which producers may select: agave, corn sweetener, corn syrup, high-fructose corn syrup, dextrose, fruit juice concentrates, honey, lactose, maltose, malt syrup, maple syrup, molasses, cane juice, cane syrup, and sucrose to name a few. Anyone looking merely for 'sugar' in the labeling may read right over them.

Sugar is highly appealing to us, well beyond the morning rush, and evidence in humans shows that sugar and sweetness can induce feelings of reward and craving much like cocaine.[67] Both human and animal studies have demonstrated that in some brains the consumption of sugar-rich food or drink primes the release of euphoric endorphins and dopamine in a manner similar to some drugs and that sugar can cause cravings and withdrawal symptoms.[68] This explains why it's so challenging to cut back or stop eating sugar entirely and also explains the great incentive food producers have to add as much sugar as possible to our food to keep us hooked and coming back for more.

This global high-sugar diet could not have existed before industrialization and the introduction of large-scale food-processing.[69] Before commercial mass production, our primary source of a concentrated sugar would have been honey, and this would naturally have had limited availability due to seasonality. Also, acquiring honey in the wild would have taken effort, and this natural scarcity would have limited how much we consumed.

The Prophet ﷺ, like the rest of us, liked sweet foods including honey,[70] and Allah tells us of the healing properties of honey in the Quran:

> *There comes forth from their bellies a drink of varying color wherein is healing for men. Verily, in this is indeed a sign for people who think. (Quran, 16:69)*

The Prophet ﷺ, did not have access to refined sugar as we know it today and took the sweet things he did eat in small portions. While our bodies can generally handle sugar in small quantities, we cannot handle sugar in the large quantities that we now consume. Reducing the amount of sugar we eat is key to gaining health and preventing sugar-related illnesses, of which there are many. Increasing awareness of where it is hidden in our food is the first step, followed by taking measures to reduce the amount we eat.

Sugar is not an essential nutrient; unlike plants, people don't actually 'need' it at all, so the FDA identifies no 'recommended daily allowance'. Rather, nutrition experts offer safe 'upper limit' guidelines of 6 or 9 teaspoons per day for women and men, respectively. Personally, I would recommend less if we are to more closely align our diet with the way the Prophet ﷺ ate. If you think only about the granulated sugar you might add to your tea and coffee, that limit might seem quite reasonable, but, once you start factoring in the sugar in all the processed food, that limit becomes a lot more challenging. Shifting back to a whole food diet, eating food the way the Prophet ﷺ ate and limiting our sugar to natural sources like honey, dates, and fruit, while minding our portion sizes, means that we also automatically reduce our sugar intake and reduce the harm that sugar does to our body.

Action Points

1. Sugar Watch: start checking your labels, looking for sugar in all its forms and paying particular attention to portion sizes.

2. Sugar Alert: pay special attention whenever you see the words 'Low Fat' as it often translates to 'High Sugar'.

3. Avoid HFCS in soda and other processed food.

4. Avoid beet sugar in processed food.

5. Use natural sweeteners (like honey, maple syrup, molasses) in small portions and remember that sugar is sugar. Just because it's natural, that doesn't mean it's ok to eat it in large quantities. A single portion of honey or similar natural sweetener is 1 tsp.

6. Limit or avoid fruit juices: these provide concentrated fructose, none of the fiber of the whole fruit and are easy to overconsume. Consider orange juice: a single glass is made from 4-5 oranges. None of us would eat 5 oranges in one go, but it is easy to drink a glass of juice and get all that sugar in one hit. Also, remember that often fruit juice may have 'fruit juice concentrate' added, raising the sugar content of the drink while still allowing producers to label it 'pure fruit juice'. If you insist on fruit juice, dilute it with water and have it at the same time as a meal to avoid blood sugar spikes.

7. Most of us need a sugar boost on occasion, for example after fasting. Following the example of the Prophet ﷺ, we can find that boost wrapped in a package of fiber and nutrients in the form of dried fruit likes dates or raisins or in fresh whole fruit.

Chapter 12

Honey

Honey is a blessed food that was loved by the Prophet ﷺ and is mentioned in both the Quran[71] and sunnah[72] as a food with incredible healing properties. In the time of the Prophet ﷺ, honey would have been one of the few primary sources of natural sugar. It would have been natural, raw and mostly seasonal, as bees would collect nectar when plants made it available.

The ever-increasing demand for honey has meant that producers are continually trying to make more, for less, to supply the booming market and boost profits. This has led to some commercial producers engaging in less-than-ethical practices such as exposing honey bees to sugar water or high fructose corn syrup instead of natural nectar and continuing to sell that honey to consumers as 'natural' since sugar and syrup originate from natural sugar cane and corn. Some products sold as honey contain pure honey only as part of the ingredient list, the rest being 'honey-flavored' sugar syrup, yet unaware consumers may not think to check the label, just assuming that what they are buying is the 'real' thing. Honey has also been affected by our use of pesticides; some of these chemicals are ending up in the honey we eat. Neonicotinoids, in particular, when sprayed on plants that are then pollinated by bees, have been detected in honey samples from around the world.[73] Commercially-produced honey is very different in composition to the natural raw honey of pre-modern diets and of the time of the Prophet ﷺ. Even 'pure and natural' honey may often have been refined and pasteurized before it hits the supermarket shelves a process which destroys most of the beneficial healing properties mentioned in the Quran and sunnah.

Action Points:

- Honey: choose raw, organic honey over processed honey to enjoy the beautiful healing benefits of this blessed food.

- Check your labels and be particularly cautious of anything that reads 'honey-flavored'.

Chapter 13

Artificial Sweeteners

Artificial sweeteners are sugar substitutes that taste sweet but, unlike natural sweeteners, generally have few or no calories. Having been designed in a lab, they can be several hundred times sweeter than sugar, so very little is needed to get a similar sweet taste, therefore they have been widely marketed as 'ideal diet food': a way to get your sweet fix while avoiding high-calorie sugar and HFCS. Artificial sweeteners also became popular because they allowed diabetics to enjoy food they hadn't been able to eat. Commercial producers have jumped on the bandwagon of the booming diet food industry, and the number of food products containing non-caloric artificial sweeteners has sky-rocketed in the last 15 years. There's no shortage of variety in the sweetener market, and many of these chemical sweeteners are heavily used in commercially produced food. Unfortunately, artificial sweeteners come with their own set of concerns including several potentially undesirable side effects, especially for those who are sensitive.

The origins of these sugar substitutes also raise eyebrows. **Saccharin**, the first artificial sweetener, was discovered in 1879 quite bizarrely by Johns Hopkins researcher Constantine Fahlberg while he was working on coal tar derivatives.[74] We can only wonder what it was about coal tar that made him think, 'hey, we could eat this!' Saccharin is about 300 times sweeter than sugar, and its discovery marked the beginning of the artificial sweetener industry.

Many decades later in 1937, a second chemical sweetener, **cyclamate,** was discovered and both were labeled GRAS (generally recognized as safe) by the Food and Drug Administration. In 1969, however, the FDA banned cyclamate because of concerns over its potential to cause cancer, which led to growing concerns over saccharin's safety. By 1977, the FDA announced a saccharin ban as well – to the chagrin of its loyal consumers. Following protests, saccharin ended up staying on the market, though a warning label was added, only to be removed in 2000. Studies have also refuted the link between cyclamate and cancer and cyclamate is still sold in around 50 countries.[75]

A third artificial sweetener, **aspartame,** was discovered in 1965. A chemical compound about 200 times sweeter than sugar, aspartame was finally approved by the FDA in 1981 for dry food only, then as a general sweetener in 1996. In 1984, Monsanto bought the brand and renamed it NutraSweet.[76] Though there have not been enough long-term studies to determine conclusive links, the sweetener is suspected of a long list of troublesome side effects including cancer, seizures, headaches, depression, attention deficit hyperactivity disorder (ADHD), dizziness, weight gain, birth defects, lupus, Alzheimer's disease and multiple sclerosis (MS).[77]

Neither health concerns nor bizarre origins have hindered the patenting of additional artificial sweeteners. **Sucralose**, for one, was discovered by a graduate student working for Tate & Lyle in 1979 who, for whatever reason, decided to substitute chlorine for three of sucrose's hydroxyl groups, and voila, one of the most popular sweeteners today came into chemical existence. Approved in 1999, Sucralose has proven to be a very profitable product line for its manufacturers.[78]

One the newest kids on the block, **neotame**, was developed by NutraSweet and approved in 2002. Neotame is the most potent sweetener on the market, with 7,000 times the sweetness of sucrose.[79] It's clear that artificial sweeteners truly embody their name. Artificial and manmade, they are now widely used in commercially processed food and feature prominently in the diet food industry, with those trying to lose weight turning to synthetic sweeteners to avoid sugar and HFCS. If they truly pulled their weight as diet foods, their suspected side effects would potentially be easier to overlook. What is most surprising, though, is that several studies suggest your diet soda actually makes you put on weight rather than lose it. As current data suggests that artificial sweeteners are positively linked to weight gain in both adults and children, we may ironically be sabotaging our efforts to lose weight by reaching for diet soda and low-fat, sugar-free products.[80]

Rather than risking our health and waistline by eating chemical sweeteners that didn't exist in the time of the Prophet ﷺ, using natural sweeteners such as honey, molasses, date sugar or maple syrup, in small portions is a more healthful option. For those with diabetes or any blood sugar conditions, explore the more natural non-sugar options available such as stevia and monk fruit.

ACTION POINTS:

- Check your labels for artificial sweeteners and avoid them where possible.

- Avoid all 'diet' foods.

- Choose natural sweeteners like honey, molasses, maple syrup, date syrup or sugar, over artificial sweeteners.

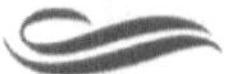

Chapter 14

Grains

There are several references to whole grains in the sunnah, including to barley and wheat,[81] among others. Grains are packed with essential nutrients, and many of the healthiest communities around the world include grains as part of a healthy diet. Studies have shown that a higher intake of whole grains is associated with 'a lower risk of cardiovascular disease and cancer, as well as death from respiratory diseases, infectious diseases, diabetes, and all non-cardiovascular, non-cancer causes.'[82] A diet that includes a higher proportion of whole grains compared to non-whole grains is associated with reducing the risk of Type 2 Diabetes in men[83] and studies have clearly shown that a combination of diet and lifestyle, particularly eating a mostly plant-based diet, with an emphasis on legumes, whole grains, vegetables, fruits, nuts, and seeds, limiting meat and animal products, is effective in preventing and managing Type 2 Diabetes.[84] This style of eating very much aligns with the diet of the Prophet ﷺ as we know it.

So, if the Prophet ﷺ ate grains, and science supports the health benefits of grains, how do we reconcile this with the trending low-carb, 'grain-free' movement that we see all around us? To understand how grains can be a part of a healthy whole food diet, and where and why some are best avoided, we have to look at how these foods have traditionally been eaten in comparison to how the majority of grains are eaten in the Standard Modern Diet (SMD). Whole grains don't feature much in the Standard Modern Diet. Rather, the majority of grains we are eating have been refined, and food items such as white rice, snow-white flour products and grain by-products like high fructose corn syrup make up a large percentage of our daily calories. We also tend to over consume these on top of even possibly overconsuming 'healthy' food. In addition to this, unlike traditional cultures in which grain soaking, sprouting or fermentation is common, we seldom prepare grains before we eat them. Regardless of how we eat them, wholegrains, just like all other healthy food, need to be eaten in reasonable portions.

WHOLEGRAINS VS. UNREFINED GRAINS VS. REFINED GRAINS

Refined grains have not actually been around very long. In the late 19th century, industrialized roller mills were invented, and this completely transformed the way we processed grains. Refining seemed like a good idea at the time. By removing the bran and germ, it was possible to dramatically increase the shelf life of products containing flour. Longer shelf life meant it was easier to transport and could sit for longer before going bad. What producers didn't know at the time was that during the process, while gaining shelf live, grains lost *most* of their essential nutrients and health benefits.

Whole grains in their original form contain three parts: bran, germ and endosperm. The bran is loaded with fiber, B vitamins, iron, copper, zinc, magnesium, antioxidants and phytochemicals. The germ contains vitamin E, B vitamins, phytochemicals, antioxidants and healthy fats. The endosperm is the interior part of the grain and contains carbohydrates and protein, as well as a small amount of vitamins and minerals. When a grain is refined, the milling process separates the bran and germ from the endosperm. It's this interior part that makes up the yummy, white refined products that we have all come to love so much in bread, pastries, cookies and cakes as well as white rice. Nutrient content aside, without bran and fiber to slow down the breakdown of starch into glucose, refined grain products cause sharp spikes in blood sugar rather than a steady rise, as with whole grains. This same fiber, when present, helps lower cholesterol and aids digestion.[85]

In the time of the Prophet ﷺ, there was no 'white flour' of today's standards, meaning flour that has been bleached with chemicals to give it its consistently snowy white hue. In the time of the Prophet ﷺ, milling was much more basic.

> *Narrated Abu Hazim: that he asked Sahl, "Did you use white flour during the lifetime of the Prophet ﷺ?" Sahl replied, "No." Hazim asked, "Did you use to sift barley flour?" He said, "No, but we used to blow off the husk (of the barley)." (Sahih Bukhari)* [86]

Fermenting, Sprouting, Soaking

Traditional cultures have also typically prepared their wholegrains before eating them by either fermenting, sprouting or soaking them making them easier to digest and to make the nutrients more available.

Pesticides, GM and Other Chemicals

A lot of the grains eaten today have been heavily sprayed with pesticides, and this pesticide residue can end up on our plates. Also, some grains, like corn, are genetically modified. It is also common for chemicals to be used during the processing of grain in some countries, as in the case of chlorine-treated cake flour and bromide in bread flour.

Growing Sensitivity to Wheat (And Other Gluten Grains)

'Gluten' has been labeled public enemy number two by the health food industry, with sugar still holding first place. As a result, 'gluten-free' has become a major selling point for the industry. It is somewhat perplexing that we are seeing a growing sensitivity to wheat and other gluten-containing grains globally. The thing about gluten is that it is inflammatory; and it has been shown to damage internal organs and tissues on contact[87] but why there is a quickly growing sensitivity to a grain that we have eaten for thousands of years is not 100% clear. For those with a disease called Celiac, gluten is particularly harmful, but what about the large percentage of people who suffer from less severe reactions to wheat like gas, bloating and skin problems or who only struggle with some gluten-containing grains, only some of the time? And why can cutting wheat out of a diet help with auto-immune conditions and other such ailments? How do we make sense of this phenomenon when wheat was eaten in the time of the Prophet ﷺ, traditional cultures have been eating wheat for thousands of years and, in many places, populations are tucking into wheat and wheat products without any issue?

The answers are not 100% clear, but there are many theories. Some say it's about breeding. Some wheat has been bred (not genetically modified, only bred) in such a way that we are less able to digest it. Others say it is not so much about the wheat but the pesticides that are sprayed on the crops while they are growing and then again during storage. Personal accounts of people who struggle to eat bread and other wheat products in the US but find they can munch their way around European bakeries without any issue, much to their gastronomical delight, gives some credence to the theory that it might have something to do with geography, though it doesn't clarify why. Yet others say that bread, mainly bread that is commercially-produced in the US, is loaded with well over a dozen ingredients, unlike traditional homemade bread, which contains only three. Or, perhaps the bread isn't what's to blame; a compromised digestive system is another explanation for the growing sensitivity to wheat and other gluten grains.

The truth is that nobody knows with 100% certainty precisely why there is a growing sensitivity. What *is* clear is that many people do benefit from limiting or removing gluten-containing grains from their diet, if not permanently then at least for a period while they heal their gut and body. Especially in the case of any form of gluten sensitivity, choosing to eat non-gluten whole grains is a better option to promote health.

ACTION POINTS:
- Replace refined grain products with whole grains.
- Avoid GM grains.
- Try to avoid non-organic grains due to pesticides.
- If choosing bread, try to find natural 3-ingredient bread. Avoid commercial bread and choose sourdough or sprouted grain bread as the best choices.

- Soak, sprout or ferment grains before eating them. Soak grains at least overnight with water combined with yogurt, buttermilk, lemon juice, whey or cider vinegar to reduce the phytic acid in the grain.[88] Sprouted flour is available at many supermarkets and, if you are keen to get into fermenting, there are several excellent books that will help you get started.

- Avoid grains containing gluten if you are sensitive to them. If you're not sure, take a break from them and see how you feel.

WHOLE GRAIN OPTIONS

While bread is often associated with wheat, there are actually numerous types of grain, as the following list shows. (Some are technically seeds, like quinoa, but I have included them in this list anyway due to their common usage as grains.)

Amaranth	Kamut	Spelt
Barley	Millet	Teff
(Brown) Rice & others	Quinoa	Triticale
Buckwheat	Rye	Wheat
Bulgur	Oat	Wild Rice
Corn	Sorghum	

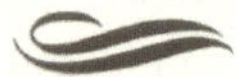

Chapter 15

Oils and Fats

The Prophet ﷺ ate natural fats such as olive oil, full-fat milk, dried yoghurt and butter, as well as meat which naturally contains fat. Alhamdullilah, these were completely natural and organic sources of dietary fat, and we need not be afraid of them. Allah, in all His wisdom, created our bodies so that they know what to do with and even require natural fats. Your brain is the fattiest organ in your body, and healthy fat is an integral part of a health-promoting diet. The problem of being overweight is not likely a result of good fat. In fact, because of our fear of fat instilled by the 'health food industry', which told us for years that all fat was bad, we aren't getting *enough* of the good fat.

Olive oil, for example, which has been proven time and again to be so heart healthy, is mentioned in both the Quran and sunnah.

And a tree (olive) that springs forth from Mount Sinai, that grows oil and (it is a) relish for the eaters. (Quran 23:20)

> *The Prophet ﷺ said, "Season (your food) with olive oil and anoint yourselves with it, for it comes from a blessed tree." (Sunan Ibn Majah)*[89]

Other natural fats are mentioned as well, such as that the Prophet ﷺ ate dried yogurt and dairy butter.[90]

The type of fat and its quality are important, as not all fats are health promoting. Good fats are good for you. The problem we are facing with oils and fat is that our modern diets are loaded with fats that are unhealthy and in excess, and many of the fats we are eating have further been damaged or contain toxins.

Excess Vegetable Oils

Think of Ramadan, and what comes to mind? Deep fried food! Yet, our love of oil cooking is relatively new, certainly not from the sunnah, and the quantity of oil we eat, notably vegetable oil, has increased dramatically since the time of the Prophet ﷺ. In the last 100 years or so alone, there has been a staggering increase in the amount of vegetable oils used. This is the result of oil seed production being industrialized so that vegetable oils are now mass produced. This overproduction has led to overconsumption. When we overconsume refined oil, we tend to overconsume refined grain along with it, as in the case of much deep fried food – a double whammy. Whereas quality fats in moderation do not 'make us fat', this style of overconsumption of unhealthy fats produces a range of health problems, including weight gain and inflammation.

This excess consumption has thrown healthy ratios of fats out of sync. Historically, we would have eaten a lot less omega 6 vegetable oil, most of which would have come from whole food like nuts and seeds in their whole form, and our diets would have been higher in omega 3 fatty acids. Excess omega 6 oils are linked to increased inflammation in our bodies, and often, amazingly, when people reduce vegetable oil consumption, a wide variety of unexplained aches and pains subside.

GM Oils

Many of the oil used in cooking and in commercially processed food is made from GM soy, corn, and canola. If the label does not mention 'GMO-free', it is likely GM in origin.

Trans Fats

We were told that butter was bad for us and margarine was good and even that it was the key to a healthy heart, but the truth about margarine revealed itself. It turns out that the trans fats in margarine have a terrible effect when it comes to heart health, exactly the issue it was long said to improve. The industrial process of hydrogenating fats involves turning an unsaturated liquid fat into a solid fat by adding hydrogen. This gives oil a longer shelf life. Unfortunately, the process can also produce trans-fatty acids (TFAs) which have been linked to cardiovascular disease, adverse lipid effects, increased inflammation and possibly the worsening of insulin sensitivity.[91] Some scientists warned that trans fats were unsafe, but it took the food industry some time to listen. Only relatively recently, in 2013, did the FDA conclude that trans fats are *not* 'generally recognized as safe' (GRAS) in food.[92]

Fortunately, trans fats have already been banned in some countries, but they are still available and widely used in other countries. Many companies in the US no longer use them, as public opinion has changed to the point that 'NO trans fats' has become a selling point. Unfortunately, these fats do still sneak their way into many commercial products like microwave popcorn, packaged pies, frozen pizza, stick margarine, ready-made frostings, commercial baked products and coffee creamers. Trans fats are also still very commonly used in India, Pakistan and the Middle East and both Vanaspati ghee (vegetable ghee) and margarine contain a high proportion of trans fats. Several studies have shown an association between TFA consumption and increased risk of cardiovascular disease (CVD), and it's been suggested that, in countries like Pakistan with high rates of cardiovascular disease, vegetable ghee might be partly to blame. Banning trans fats in the Middle East and Asia could be key to significantly reducing the risk of heart disease if Denmark's example is anything to go by. The country saw an almost 50% reduction in the number of deaths from coronary heart disease over 20 years after banning trans fats.[93]

Purity of Oils

Olive oil has long been appreciated, but since modern consumers have cottoned on to its health benefits, it is seriously big business, and where there is money to be made, there is always the risk of fraud and corruption. When we buy olive oil, we generally assume it is indeed olive oil. We trust that we are getting what we pay for and that it's the real deal, but several recent scandals have exposed certain countries' books not tallying up. They are exporting more olive oil than they produce. The purity of olive oil and other oils is also increasingly questionable, with some unscrupulous producers mixing in cheaper oils and adding flavors yet selling the oil as pure.

DAMAGED OILS

Most of us are aware, sometimes from our own attempts to multi-task while cooking, that oils have a smoking point. When they are overheated to the point of smoking, they become damaged, producing compounds which can be harmful to our health.

GENERAL EXCESS

Because we have so much available to us all the time, it is easy for us to overconsume fats and oils especially when they are hidden in processed foods.

FATS IN MEAT, FISH AND OTHER FOOD

Healthy fats can also be found in a wide variety of other food including meat, eggs, dairy and fish, a blessed food mentioned in the Quran. Many sources of fish, such as salmon, mackerel and sardines, are loaded with the wonderfully health-promoting omega 3. Seeds such as flax and chia are packed with healthy fats and even certain fruit and vegetables, like avocadoes and little known purslane, are an excellent source of healthy fats.

DIFFERENT FROM THE TIME OF THE PROPHET ﷺ

In the time of the Prophet ﷺ, there was no excess of vegetable oil nor any trans fats, just pure, simple, natural fats the way Allah made them in the form that our bodies know how to use, and there was also limited availability and variety. Nowadays, it has become a lot more complicated to navigate oils and fats because we just have so much choice and it is also being snuck into processed food in large quantities. Supermarket shelves display dozens of bottles of every type, from olive to coconut, to walnut, almond, macadamia, sesame, peanut, corn, soy, canola, sunflower and more. Each of these has different properties, different shelf lives, different smoking points, different potential of being damaged. We now need to study up just to select and use oils.

In the time of the Prophet ﷺ, variety was limited, and any nuts and seeds that were available would likely have been consumed whole (along with their fiber content) more often than pressed or processed. He ﷺ did not have to navigate a sea of oil choices. He ﷺ ate what was available. The Prophet ﷺ ate meat, butter and dried yogurt and drank milk, all of which have natural saturated fat and make up part of a healthy diet in moderation. As with many foods, it is not often the case that more is better. Natural fats are beneficial – in balanced amounts. We do not need enormous quantities of them, just as we do not require enormous quantities of any other food. In the time of the Prophet ﷺ, supply of animal fat was naturally limited due to naturally limited availability. Unlike many of us, the Prophet ﷺ did not eat meat daily. He also encouraged the use of olive oil.[94]

Action Points

Avoid/Limit

- Trans fats including margarine, vegetable 'ghee' and shortening
- Excess vegetable oils (as excess can lead to inflammation)
- GM oils: soy, canola, corn

Making the Best Oil and Fat Choices

- Olive oil is the superstar of the oils. Buy organic if you can. If not, research a trusted source in your country. Olive oil is good for salads and can be safely used to sauté food.

- Use oils, other than olive oil, sparingly. Instead, get your fats from whole food (e.g., sunflower seeds vs. sunflower oil, avocados vs. avocado oil, walnuts vs. walnut oil)

- If you are using oils to cook, don't heat then to temperatures above their smoking point as they oxidize and are no longer healthy.

- Different oils can be tasty and health promoting, but you don't need a wide variety of oils to be healthy. Purchasing large amounts is likely to result in either overconsumption or waste.

- Keep oil in dark glass bottles in cool places, and buy small quantities to prevent them going rancid. This is particularly important for heat-sensitive oils like flax.

- Butter, dairy ghee and tallow are all excellent fat choices for cooking as they are safe at high heat. Try sourcing organic from grass-fed, pasture-raised animals.

- Include healthy fats in your diet such as nuts, seeds, olives, avocado, fish, eggs, meat and full fat (organic, pasture-raised) dairy.

Chapter 16

Milk and Dairy

And indeed, for you in grazing livestock is a lesson. We give you drink from what is in their bellies - between excretion and blood - pure milk, palatable to drinkers. (Quran 16:66)

Milk is considered a whole food, providing an amazing 18 out of 22 essential nutrients, subhan Allah. It contains more calcium, magnesium, phosphorus, potassium, zinc, and protein per calorie than any other food in a typical diet. Milk can help control appetite, it is beneficial for bone development and it may help prevent heart disease,[95] but there is a downside to milk, too. For one, many people are allergic to milk or have a sensitivity to it. It can worsen certain skin conditions like eczema, and excess calcium from milk and other foods may increase the risk of prostate cancer.[96]

But the commercially-produced milk most of us drink today is a far cry from the milk that was available in the time of the Prophet ﷺ, when the Quran was revealed. Regarding whether *today's* milk is a health food, there are some factors to consider. Firstly, we need to look at the source of the milk and how it is processed. Natural, organic, raw whole milk from healthy cows pastured on natural pesticide-free grass is vastly different from commercially produced milk from cows kept in confinement, implanted with growth hormones, given routine antibiotics and fed a diet of GM corn heavily sprayed with pesticides. Commercial milk is also homogenized for consistency and pasteurized using heat to kill any harmful bacteria, which are more likely in the context of mass production. Not only is natural milk better for the environment, it is nutritionally superior, with more antioxidants and, on average, 68% more omega 3 fatty acids. What's more, organic cheese can have up to twice as many nutrients as conventional cheese.[97]

Aside from nutritional quality, we also need to consider the quantity we consume. Too much dairy, like too much of any food, can be harmful to our health. Moreover, it's important to remember that just because a particular food benefits many people, that does not mean that it is healthy for everyone. If you are lactose intolerant (sensitive to the naturally occurring sugar in milk) or have any other allergy or sensitivity to milk, or if it increases inflammation in your body, then milk – organic, raw or otherwise – is not a health food for you. Studies also suggest that a particular portion of the human population loses the ability to digest milk as they get older. This may further explain why so many people struggle with the Standard Modern Diet that is so high in dairy.

About Hormones in Milk

"It really depends on how you look at the science. Many industry-funded studies show no risk, but there are independent studies that suggest a potential <u>cancer</u> risk from hormones in milk." [98]

Many countries have now banned the use of hormones in milk production because of its questionable safety and potential risk of long-term side effects. While our ideal may be to have raw organic milk as it was drunk in the time of the Prophet ﷺ, this may not be possible for most of us. Raw milk is not easy to come by, partially because much caution is required to ensure that it comes from a safe source, as raw milk can carry diseases. As a second-best option, organic whole milk from grass-fed, pasture-raised cows is a good alternative. If commercial dairy is your only option, it's best to limit the amount you consume and boost your calcium intake by way of other natural whole foods.

ACTION POINTS

- Choose organic milk and dairy from pasture-raised, grass-fed animals.

- If you have a safe source of raw organic milk, this milk is closest to the way the Prophet  would have consumed it, but, I emphasize again, the source MUST be clean and safe if you are drinking it raw.

Chapter 17

Meat

And the grazing livestock He has created for you; in them is warmth and [numerous] benefits, and from them you eat. (Quran 16:5)

That [has been commanded], and whoever honors the sacred ordinances of Allah - it is best for him in the sight of his Lord. And permitted to you are the grazing livestock, except what is recited to you. So avoid the uncleanliness of idols and avoid false statement. (Quran 22:30)

Verily Allah has enjoined goodness to everything; so when you kill, kill in a good way and when you slaughter, slaughter in a good way. So every one of you should sharpen his knife, and let the slaughtered animal die comfortably. (Sahih Muslim)[99]

Alhamdulillah, Allah has provided food in the form of animal flesh that is incredibly nutritious, and He has made it permissible for us, but it's important to understand that, before and after slaughter, a lot can go wrong. Because meat production has been industrialized and continues to change so much, it's necessary to differentiate between the various types of meat that may end up on our dinner plate.

TYPES OF MEAT

1. Conventional: red meat (lamb, beef, goat, etc.) and white meat (poultry) is generally raised in large feedlots with animals fed a diet high in commercially-produced grain. They are also commonly given antibiotics and sometimes growth hormones.

2. Processed: any meat that is subjected to processing methods beyond butchering, for example, sandwich meat, hot dogs and other sausages.

3. Organic: grass-fed, pasture-raised red meat and pasture-raised poultry.

Of these types of meat, number 3 is the closest to the meat produced in the time of the Prophet ﷺ. First, let's take a more careful look at red meat, then we'll look at poultry in the next section.

MEAT HAS CHANGED

The practice of feeding grain (mostly corn) to livestock became popular after technological developments made mass production of grain possible. Before 1850, almost all cattle in the US were free-range or pasture fed, and they were generally slaughtered at around 4-5 years of age. With the introduction of feedlots and the science of fattening cattle quickly, farmers were thereafter able to ready a full-grown steer for slaughter in just 2 years, but the meat was 'marbled'. Unlike grain fed animals, pasture-raised animals have meat that looks more like that of wild game. Less than a century later, in the 1950s, feedlots appeared that could hold up to 100,000 cattle, all ready for slaughter in just 14 months. Today, meat from grain-fed animals makes up about 99% of all beef eaten in the US.[100] This massive production is a relatively very recent development and did not exist even 200 years ago, let alone in the time of the Prophet ﷺ.

COMMERCIALLY PRODUCED MEAT MAY BE CONTAMINATED WITH HORMONES AND PESTICIDES

The FDA has approved a number of steroid drugs for use over the last 70 years, including natural estrogen, progesterone, testosterone, and their synthetic versions. These steroids aim to speed up the animal's growth rate and their ability to convert their food into meat and are administered either as pellets or implants placed under the skin of the animal's ear.[101] This modern reality is eerily reminiscent of, though not necessarily connected to, the shaitan's promised corruption, as documented in the Quran, in which he says that

"I will mislead them, and I will arouse in them [sinful] desires, and I will command them so they will slit the ears of cattle, and I will command them so they will change the creation of Allah.' And whoever takes Satan as an ally instead of Allah has certainly sustained a clear loss" (Quran 4:119).

Commercial meat can also contain pesticide residue, even so much as exceeds safety thresholds, as was discovered in one study of cattle tissue, suggesting possible health risks for consumers, particularly children.[102]

COMMERCIAL MEAT HAS A MASSIVELY NEGATIVE EFFECT ON THE ENVIRONMENT

All these cattle have to be fed, and it takes a considerable amount of grain to produce meat. It's estimated that it takes about 15 pounds of grain to produce just two pounds of industrial beef. According to David Pimentel, professor of ecology in Cornell University's College of Agriculture and Life Sciences, "If all the grain currently fed to livestock in the United States were consumed directly by people, the number of people who could be fed would be nearly 800 million."[103] Like the cattle it feeds, this grain is commercially mass-produced and requires large amounts of pesticides and fertilizers. According to a Times article, *Getting real about the high price of cheap food,* more than 10 million tons of fertilizers are used for corn alone – and nearly 23 million for crops overall. Waste and chemicals have to go somewhere; as they say, all roads lead to the ocean, and run-off from these farms has significantly contributed to the 'dead zone' in the Gulf of Mexico, a "6,000-sq.-mi. area that has almost no oxygen and therefore almost no sea life." The article also states that, worse, there are around 400 similar dead zones in water bodies around the world.[104]

ETHICS

The way animals are treated in commercial food production raises some serious ethical considerations for us as Muslims. Kind treatment of animals is part of our deen and additionally results in reward from Allah, according to the sunnah, while cruel treatment can justify punishment.

> *The Messenger of Allah ﷺ happened to pass by a camel whose belly was sticking to its back (because of hunger), whereupon he said, "Fear Allah in respect of these mute (animals). Ride them while they are fit, and slaughter them and eat their meat when they are fit." (Abu Dawud)*[105]

> *The Prophet ﷺ said, "A woman entered the (Hell) Fire because of a cat which she had tied, neither giving it food nor setting it free to eat from the vermin of the earth." (Sahih Bukhari)*[106]

We may not be able to walk into a commercial feedlot and make them change the way they treat animals, but every time we buy food, we essentially vote with our money, and there's nothing that speaks louder than cash to commercial producers. One person refusing to buy may not have any effect, but 1.8 billion people making a change certainly would. Choosing quality over quantity could literally transform the entire industry, saving millions of animals from a life of misery and dramatically reducing the negative impact of excess meat production on our planet, all while allowing us to enjoy greater health and seek Allah's reward for actively supporting kind treatment to animals by refusing to participate in cruelty.

IS MEAT A HEALTH FOOD?

On top of all the issues surrounding conventional meat are rumors that red meat is not healthy and should be avoided. There are never-ending debates about whether meat is a health food at all. It's true that consumption of processed meat and overconsumption of meat in general have been associated through studies with a higher risk of cardiovascular disease, cancer, and death from disease.[107] Another study specified that it was processed meat, not red meat in general, that was linked to a higher rate of diabetes and cardiovascular disease[108] although observational studies have linked high consumption of red meat with colorectal cancer.[109] Yet other studies suggest that it is the way meat is cooked, and the harmful compounds that form in the cooking process, especially cooking involving high heat such as pan frying or grilling, that results in increased risk.[110]

Alhamdulillah, as Muslims, the answer to the question of whether or not meat is healthy is simple. Allah has made meat permissible on the condition that it is halal, and we know that the Creator would not permit us to eat something that was not generally beneficial to us. However, in connection with such permission, we have also been given guidance on limitations. If we look at the example of the Prophet ﷺ, he did not eat meat daily and certainly not multiple times a day. There was also no processed meat in the time of the Prophet ﷺ and animals were raised naturally. If we follow his example and choose to eat meat the way Allah designed it – organic and pasture-raised – and in small quantities, as the Prophet ﷺ did, then meat is an incredibly nutritious and health-promoting food.

It is also not an obligation for us to eat meat. As we see in the sunnah of the Prophet ﷺ, if he did not prefer something, he did not eat it, but nor did he criticize food.[111] Based on that example, if a Muslim chooses not to eat meat or any other halal food out of preference, that's a personal decision to be respected.

COST OF ORGANIC

It's true that organic meat costs more than commercially produced meat, but, if we can adopt a principle of quality over quantity, we stand to benefit immensely. By reducing our meat consumption for the sake of following the example of the Prophet ﷺ, for the benefit of our health, and by choosing not to support mass producers who raise animals with no quality of life, we can use the money saved on quantity of meat to increase the quality, earn reward and gain health benefits at the same time.

ACTION POINTS

1. Choose quality over quantity. Choose organic meat where possible.

2. Reduce meat consumption in general. You could start with one meat-free day every week where you try out a new vegetarian recipe. Reduce the portion sizes of meat in each meal.

3. Limit or avoid char-grilled meat.

4. Cook meat slowly over a longer period on lower temperatures. Try out a crock pot.

5. If you cook on high heat, avoid burning the meat.

Chapter 18

Chicken

Chicken is a firm favorite for most of us, with dishes ranging from curries to stir-fries, roasts, nuggets, burgers, sausages, kebabs and more featuring on our dinner plates. It's tasty, and, for the most part, it's affordable, but where does our chicken come from, and how are farmers producing chickens at such low prices?

Chicken does come at a price, it's just not one that is immediately apparent. The global demand for chicken is massive, and the ever-increasing demand for cheap and abundant chicken meat has completely transformed the face of meat production. Over the last 80 years, production techniques have changed dramatically as farmers have looked for ways to increase the weight of chickens while decreasing production time, fulfilling the voracious appetite of meat eaters worldwide. In 1925, a broiler chicken would take a little over 110 days to go from being hatched to being ready for slaughter and would weigh in at a final 2.75 lbs (1.25 kg), more or less. By 2010, commercial broiler chickens weighing 5.5 lbs (2.5 kg) each were ready for slaughter in just 47 days in the US and 42 days in Europe.[112]

Commercial broilers grow quickly, saving producers both time and money. They are raised in vast sheds that are often windowless, with many chickens never seeing the light of day in their short lives. There can be up to 20,000 birds in a single shed, and the birds are generally fed a diet of commercial grain aimed to fatten them up as quickly as possible. Litter scatters the shed's floor which is usually not cleaned during the lifetime of the birds. When litter gets wet, it can lead to contact dermatitis and lesions on the birds' bodies. These incredibly abnormal, cramped conditions can result in outbreaks of disease, so to avoid that, antibiotics are routinely added to the chickens' food.[113] Nobody likes the idea of animals being mistreated or suffering, but, sadly, this is what happens with much of commercial production. Industries are desperate to prevent consumers finding out just how their food is produced because they know that, once we know, we won't want to buy from them anymore. Toward this end, there is now what's called the 'Ag Gag' law "that criminalizes investigative journalists and animal protection advocates who take entry-level jobs at factory farms."[114] Several US states have passed or attempted to pass such a law though some courts have found the law to be unconstitutional as a violation of the First Amendment.[115]

ANTIBIOTICS AND FEED

Astoundingly, around 80% of all antibiotics sold in the US are intended for use in commercial livestock. Of these, about 70% are considered 'medically important', meaning they are antibiotics important to human beings.[116] There is increasing evidence that the use of antibiotics in animals is linked to antibiotic resistance in humans.[117] In 2015 the World Health Organization (WHO) was driven to issue a statement on this crisis-in-action, warning that antimicrobial resistance is "an increasingly serious threat to global public health that requires action across all government sectors and society."[118] Commercial chicken, like commercial beef, is also raised primarily on grain, an altogether unnatural diet that lacks many of the nutrients that a happy chicken scratching around in the dirt eating bugs and seeds would enjoy.

THEN AND NOW

In the time of the Prophet ﷺ, animals would have been raised in a natural environment as there were no mass production facilities. In contrast, the vast majority of commercial meat is now produced in mass facilities. If we want to buy a chicken that was raised in a natural environment, that grew up slowly, that pecked and scratched in the dirt, ate bugs and had a good quality of life, doing all the things chickens do, the only option we have is to pay extra and buy pasture-raised and organic. Alternatively, we can source natural chickens from a local farmer or raise and slaughter chickens ourselves.

Choosing not to eat commercial chicken is not an easy choice because, for most of us, chicken probably makes up a large percentage of our weekly meals. Chicken is versatile, tasty and affordable. When we buy it, we don't generally think about why it's so cheap. We also tend not to think about the source of the food we are buying or eating. It's easy to swallow a bowl of 10 chicken wings without a thought that those wings came from 5 live animals. It's easy to buy a pack of 8 chicken breasts, all fresh looking and vacuum sealed, without thinking that those breasts came from 4 live chickens. Making changes is a step process, and the first step is awareness of the meat industry's practices as they affect the choices available to you.

As a starting point, know your chickens:

- **Commercial Chickens** - raised in large sheds, sometimes without windows. Fed on commercial grain and often given antibiotics. This type constitutes the vast majority of chicken available today.

- **Higher Welfare Chickens** - given more space and light and allowed to express more natural behavior and grow more slowly. Limited availability.

- **Free Range Chickens** - have some access to outdoor living at least some of the time. They may still be fed commercial grain.

- **Organic Chickens** - free range and should have access to natural vegetation. Slower growing breeds are used, with a lower density of birds in living space.

THE ETHICAL CHOICE

In shaa Allah, when we choose to eat meat that is ethically sourced, we have the opportunity to earn reward for preventing the suffering of an animal.

Abu Hurayra reported that the Messenger of Allah ﷺ said, "One day a man became very thirsty while walking down the road. He came across a well, went down into it, and drank and then climbed out. In front of him, he found a dog panting, eating the dust out of thirst. The man said, 'This dog is as thirsty as I was.' He went back down into the well and filled his shoe, putting it into his mouth (in order to climb back up) and then gave the dog water. Therefore Allah thanked him and forgave him." It was said in reply, "Messenger of Allah, will we have a reward on account of animals?" He said, "There is a reward on account of every living thing." (Al-Adab Al-Mufrad)[119]

MAKING CHANGES

Making better choices is a process. Cutting out commercial meat can be challenging if it's a large part of our diet, so take it step-by-step and make the best choices you can given your circumstances and the resources available to you. If we can adopt a principle of quality over quantity, gradually reducing how much meat we eat for the sake of following the example of the Prophet ﷺ, for the benefit of our health, and choosing not to support mass producers who raise animals with no quality of life, we can use the money saved on quantity to increase the quality. Allah is Merciful, and He knows your intention, so do what you can and don't create a burden upon yourself beyond what you can manage. Small but consistent steps can make a significant difference over time. Community-wide changes can make more difference than individual- or family-level changes.

ACTION POINTS

1. Choose quality over quantity.

2. Make the best choice you can: higher welfare is better than commercially raised, free-range is better than higher welfare and organic is better than free-range. Remember, it's about progress, so set your intention and aim to take it one small step at a time.

3. Be mindful of your food source and quantities: think about where that bucket of chicken wings came from, where the 8-pack of chicken breasts came from. Remembering that the meat we

are eating came from animals that were once alive, whose entire purpose (if mass produced) was to serve our desire for always-available meat, gives us a new appreciation for what we are eating and for how much we are eating. Connecting to our food source will increase gratitude and reduce the amount we're likely to eat.

4.	Reduce meat consumption in general. You could try to have one meat-free day every week to start, each week trying out a new vegetarian recipe. Also, reduce the portion size of meat in each meal.

5.	Make meat go further. Example of how to use 1 whole chicken for 3 meals for a family of 4 using meat as a *flavor*, not the focus:

- Use chicken breasts, finely shredded, in a chicken and veg stir fry or with black beans, onion, red pepper and taco spice (served with brown rice, avocado and salsa)

- Use legs in a chicken, potato and vegetable stew or curry (cook meat then remove from the bone and shred it).

- Use the carcass – boil with onions, vegetables, herbs and spices for soup/broth and benefit from the nutrients and collagen in the bones.

6.	Limit or avoid char-grilled meat.

7.	Cook meat slowly over a longer period and on lower temperatures. Try out a crock pot.

8.	If you cook on high heat, avoid burning the meat.

Chapter 19

Eggs

Eggs had a bad reputation for a long time. In 1968, the American Heart Association, concerned about dietary cholesterol, told the population that they should eat no more than 3 eggs a week which resulted in a significant reduction in the number of eggs eaten by those with diseases and also those who were healthy. Even in undeveloped countries, the population was advised against eating eggs.

> *In 1968, the American Heart Association recommended the consumption of no more than 300 mg/day of dietary cholesterol and emphasized that no more than 3 eggs should be eaten per week, resulting in substantial reductions in egg consumption, not just by diseased populations but also by healthy individuals, and more importantly by poor communities in undeveloped counties who were advised against consuming a highly nutritious food.*[120]

Newly-released dietary guidelines have changed their tune, and eggs are no longer in the health food dog box. Rather, eggs have now been recognized as a nutritious whole food, packed with protein, fat and essential nutrients. They contain choline and are also a good source of dietary vitamin D. They're tasty, versatile and can be enjoyed alone in a variety of ways or used as part of many other dishes. Some recommendations suggest a maximum of 2–6 yolks per week. However, there is limited evidence to support this restriction and other studies, observing people eating 1-3 eggs per day, in almost all cases showed an increase in 'good' HDL cholesterol, and 'bad' LDL cholesterol remained mostly unchanged in most but in 30% of people — called hyper-responders — LDL markers do go up slightly so it seems that the answer to how many eggs it is ok to eat is that it depends on the individual and probably also on the overall make-up of an individual's diet.[121]

If you are concerned about your cholesterol or are unsure whether it is safe for you to consume eggs, please consult your GP or a naturopathic doctor to find out what the best option for you is.

Unfortunately, much like the meat industry, now that mass production of eggs is up and running, the vast majority of eggs available on the market are commercially produced by battery hens who live in terribly cramped conditions, sometimes confined in small cages not much larger than a piece of printing paper cubed. Though times may differ, battery hens live in these conditions for approximately 17 months until they are collected from farms and taken to be slaughtered because they are deemed 'no longer commercially viable' as they may be laying fewer eggs. On a positive note, an increasing number of websites are working to rehome post-commercial hens via adoption to give them a better quality of life.[122]

Most commercial hens are fed a diet consisting largely of GM grains along with additives to boost nutrient content. Ever wondered how 'omega 3 rich' eggs are achieved? Flax seed is added to the feed. Even egg yolk color is affected by what the hens eat, and producers often add ingredients, not necessarily artificial, to feed that makes the egg yolk more yellow, creating the uniform, deep yellow color we have come to associate with nutrient density and quality.

DEBEAKING

Because of the cramped conditions, debeaking (removing a portion of the beak) is common practice in the egg industry, deemed necessary to prevent hens from pecking at each other to the point of injury and even cannibalism, one of the major causes of death among commercial laying hens whose beaks have not been trimmed. Pecking is a normal chicken behavior, an instinctive way these very social animals establish order and hierarchy in groups, but it becomes an issue in the context of unnatural confinement, where hens have no outlet for their normal requirements of foraging, exploring and dustbathing. Beak trimming may cause pain (acute, chronic, or both) due to tissue damage or nerve injury.[123]

PROTECTING THE SHADY HENHOUSE

Egg producers know that consumers don't want to buy eggs produced under such inhumane conditions, and so have come up with various creative ways to make their eggs appear more wholesome and appealing. From the beautiful picture of the fat, happy-looking hen on the egg carton, which looks absolutely nothing like the actual production facility, to dazzling promises of omega 3 and other amazing nutrients or even reduced cholesterol content. Even 'vegetarian fed' has become a selling point, which is somewhat perplexing as chickens, by nature, are not vegetarian; they would ordinarily eat bugs along with seeds and other nutritious titbits they'd find while scratching around in their natural environment. If vegetarian means GM grain, then the packaging is akin to a wolf in sheep's clothing

One of the most inhumane practices is one of which consumers tend to be least aware: the routine culling of male chicks in commercial hatcheries. The Royal Society for the Prevention of Cruelty to Animals describes the process thusly:

In the egg industry, the sex of day-old chicks is determined at the hatchery. Sexing chicks (determining whether they are a hen or a rooster) requires considerable skill and is done at this very early stage to determine their fate.

If strong and healthy, the female chicks remain in the hatchery, they are grown to a suitable size and then transferred to a laying facility — which could be a caged, free-range or barn set up. Male chicks are considered an unwanted by product of egg production and are killed and disposed of shortly after birth.

Male chicks are killed for two reasons: they cannot lay eggs and they are not suitable for chicken-meat production. This is because layer hens — and

therefore their chicks — are a different breed of poultry to chickens that are bred and raised for meat production. Layer hens are bred to produce eggs whereas meat chickens are bred to grow large breast muscle and legs.

The <u>Model Code of Practice for the Welfare of Animals: Domestic Poultry</u> states that all culled or surplus newly hatched chicks that are destined for disposal must be treated as humanely as those that will be retained or sold. They must be destroyed promptly by a recommended humane method such as carbon dioxide gassing or quick maceration. Chicks must then be carefully inspected to ensure they are all are dead.

Quick maceration ensures the chick is killed within a second and, if carried out effectively and competently, this method may be considered more humane than gassing with high concentrations of carbon dioxide. Gassing results in gasping and head shaking and, depending on the mixture of gases used, it may take up to two minutes for the chick to die.

The RSPCA continues to urge the egg industry to invest in alternatives that avoid the potential for pain and suffering with current killing methods of male chicks. For example, research into alternatives to allow chick sex to be determined in the early egg incubation phase should be urgently progressed.[124]

THE NUTRITIONAL DIFFERENCE BETWEEN COMMERCIAL AND ORGANIC PASTURE-RAISED EGGS

Eggs from organic chickens raised on pasture boast three to six times the vitamin D content of conventional eggs, 66% more vitamin A, three times more vitamin E, seven times more beta-carotene, twice the omega 3 fats, 33% less cholesterol, and 25% less saturated fat.[125]

BENEFITING FROM A MORE NATURAL CHOICE

Eggs can be a wonderful part of a whole food diet, but knowing just how most eggs are produced is upsetting and frustrating, especially as eggs make up a staple part of most of our diets and many of our recipes. Organic eggs are a beautiful solution but can be expensive, at least compared to cheap conventional eggs, and may be limited in availability.

ACTION PONTS

Remember that the pretty picture on the carton is most likely not one of the actual farm and that most eggs, *unless specifically labelled otherwise,* are commercially produced. Details such as brown shell, 'cage-free' and 'antibiotic-free' are essentially meaningless. Remember, as with everything, it's a step process and we can only do what we can and choose the best options available to us given our situation and availability.

- **Commercial Eggs** – Raised in enclosures and or/cages, hens may never see the light of day, de-beaking is likely practiced and they are likely fed antibiotics and a diet high in GM grain.

- **Free Range** – Hens will have some outdoor access but there are generally no regulations on what type of outdoor access this is or the quality, de-beaking likely practiced, most likely fed antibiotics and a diet high in GM grain.

- **Vegetarian** – Hens likely fed a diet high in GM grain but they will not be fed ground animal parts which is sometimes included in animal feed. 'Vegetarian' hens may be raised in enclosures and or/cages, may never see the light of day, de-beaking is likely practiced and they are likely fed antibiotics and a diet high in GM grain.

- **Omega 3** – This simply means that the hens have food high in omega 3, such as flax seed, added to their diet. These hens may be raised in enclosures and or/cages, may never see the light of day, de-beaking is likely practiced and they are likely fed antibiotics and a diet high in GM grain.

- **Pasture-raised or grass-ranged, organic, raised without antibiotics** – This is the BEST CHOICE as it is the most natural option, as close to the way Allah made it as possible. This is the most ethical option as well.

Get Your Own Chook

Keeping chickens is becoming an increasingly popular option for conscientious egg-buyers who want a consistent supply of delicious, wholesome eggs direct from their backyard. There are several books, blogs and groups, including the Muslim Homestead Facebook page[126], where you can find out more about how to raise your own chickens.

Head to Your Local Farmers' Market

If you aren't quite ready to get your own chickens, farmers' markets can be a great option and may be less expensive than store-bought pasture-raised, organic eggs.

Connect with Others

Chances are, there are other natural food lovers in your area. They may already have their own laying hens with excess eggs to sell. They're also likely to know the best place to get fresh natural eggs in your area, so I highly recommend getting connected locally.

Chapter 20

Fish and Seafood

And it is He who subjected the sea for you to eat from it tender meat and to extract from it ornaments which you wear. And you see the ships plowing through it, and [He subjected it] that you may seek of His bounty; and perhaps you will be grateful. (Quran 16:14)

Fish is a blessing and is known to be an amazing health food, packed with protein and other beneficial nutrients, but, unfortunately in our modern times, not all fish is equal in benefit and some is associated with particular harm, either to our health or to the environment. Because of the increasing demand for fish, there has been an increase in fish farming, and, just as with commercially mass-produced meat, chicken and eggs, commercial fish farmers often feed fish unnatural high-grain diets as well as antibiotics to prevent them from getting sick in abnormally cramped environments.

Even when choosing fish from the ocean, because of the damage we have done to our environment, such fish are often contaminated with high levels of heavy metals, especially mercury. Increasingly, plastic is also an issue, with fish in the ocean ingesting microscopic plastic particles that we end up eating.

Action Points

- Choose wild-caught fish over farmed fish.

- Look for an eco-label on the package and ask where the fish came from.

- Support ocean-friendly food, and use the Seafood Watch website www.seafoodwatch.org as a guide if you are in the US. If you live outside North America, do a local search for sustainable, clean fish and seafood.

Chapter 21

Water

Water is key to our survival. It dissolves nutrients, so we can absorb them, aids metabolism, transports chemicals and nutrients throughout our body, eliminates waste, absorbs and transports heat and helps control appetite. This blessed substance is what makes up every living thing, and it keeps us alive. Allah has provided us with the greatest blessing in water.

> *Have those who disbelieved not considered that the heavens and the earth were a joined entity, and We separated them and made from water every living thing? Then will they not believe? (Quran 21:30)*

> *Water is the resource of life, the best drink there is and one of the pillars of existence. Rather it is the most important pillar of life as Allah has created every living thing from water. (Imam Ibn Al-Qayyim Al-Jauziyah, Healing with the Medicine of the Prophet ﷺ)*[127]

Purity

If you have ever tasted natural water direct from a pure source, like a mountain spring, you will know how incredible it is. Water like this is full of minerals and is clean and safe. Drinking natural water can be risky, though, if it does not come from a clean source. It can be contaminated not only with bacteria but also chemicals, pharmaceuticals and other pollution. A study carried out by the United States Geological Survey (USGS) discovered BPA (commonly used in plastic that disrupts endocrine functions if ingested), methotrexate (an immunosuppressant and cancer treatment) and the antibiotic sulfamethoxazole in ground water.[128]

Tap water may seem the safer bet to ground water, but even that comes with risks and challenges. Aside from the effects of chlorine and fluoride, since 2010, water testing has found dozens of contaminants, including heavy metals, in Americans' tap water, according to an EWG drinking water quality analysis. The quality of tap water can differ greatly from municipality to municipality and from country to country so it's worth doing some research to find out how safe your local water is for drinking and what options are available.[129]

Resource for Water Purity Assessment in the US: https://www.ewg.org/tapwater/

Commodfication of Water

Because of the issues of water safety, the sale of bottled water has sky-rocketed into a multi-billion dollar industry. The bottled water industry was valued at USD 185 billion in 2015 and is expected to reach USD 334 billion by 2023.[130] It is big business.

While the industry was still in its youth, the CEO of Nestle issued a highly controversial statement:

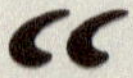

Water is, of course, the most important raw material we have today in the world. It's a question of whether we should privatize the normal water supply for the population. And there are two different

When criticized for his stance on human rights, he commented that he believed his statement has been taken out of context, but the essence of commodifying water was heard loud and clear.

As common as bottled water is today, if you were to go back even just 50 years and tell people that a time would come in the not too distant future when many people would have to purchase basic drinking water in bottles, they would never have believed you. If they did, they might at least expect such water to be high quality mineral water, not tap water that is simply run through a filtration system, as is bottled today.

As water is so vital to our health, trying to source the best possible water is also key to our health. That can be challenging. To find the best water source for you and your family, you'll need to do some local research as to what is available for you and factor in what is affordable. Find out what the water is like in your municipality. If you can afford it, a water filtration system is an excellent option. Unfortunately, water filters can be pricey and are simply not affordable for many. Something is better than nothing, in the context of drinking water, so even a water filter jug that removes chlorine is a good start, then you can work your way up based on whatever you can afford. If you are able to save up and invest in a water filter, it actually works out cheaper than buying mineral water over the course of a year, plus you save all that plastic. Another option is sourcing a local water supply. Some cities have places where you can buy filtered water by the gallon, so you save on the initial outlay of the filter while benefitting from safe and clean water.

ACTION POINTS

- The quality of water varies dramatically from place to place so you'll need to do some local research as to what is available to you and what is affordable.

- Find out what the tap water is like in your municipality.

- If you can afford it, a water filtration system is an excellent option.

- Unfortunately, water filters can be pricey and are simply not affordable for many.

- Something is better than nothing, so even a counter-top water filter jug that removes chlorine is a good start, and then work your way up based on whatever you can afford.

- If you are able to save up and invest in a water filter, it actually works out cheaper than buying mineral water over the course of a year and you also save on all that plastic.

- Another option is sourcing a local water supply. Some cities have places where you can go and buy filtered water by the gallon, so you save on the initial outlay of the water filter but still get to benefit from safe and clean water.

Chapter 22

Packaging and Cooking

PACKAGING, STORAGE AND PREPARATION

Though this book is about food, packaging necessarily pushes its way into the conversation – and not only for the way food is wrapped, labeled and marketed by producers. The *materials* used in industrial packaging and even in food storage at home, as well as food preparation, have a significant effect on our health and on our environment. In the time of the Prophet ﷺ, only natural materials were available as storage options. We are blessed with many new materials that make storage and cooking easier in our time, but some of them do present a risk to our health. We all know that plastic is a massive problem, but, alhamdulillah, this heightened awareness is leading to innovation and reform.

BPA

BPA is an endocrine disruptor that mimics estrogen and it has also been labelled 'obesogenic', meaning that is can cause obesity. BPA has been linked to heart disease, Type 2 Diabetes and, in infants born to mothers who have been exposed to BPA, a negative effect on birth weight as well as other symptoms. Studies also suggest that BPA may cause infertility in men and women, raise the risk of obesity and cause other health issues such as PCOS, asthma, abnormal liver function, worsened immune function, impaired thyroid function and premature delivery.[132] Used for years in can linings, plastic containers and plastic dishes and cups, in July 2012, the FDA finally ruled that BPA can no longer be used in sippy cups and baby bottles but have not limited its use elsewhere.[133]

PFCs (Perfluorochemicals)

PFCs are used in non-stick cookware and oil-resistant food packaging, amongst other things. Data on the effects of PFC on humans is sparse, but animal studies have linked PFCs to infant death, several types of tumors and additional toxic effects on the liver and the immune and endocrine systems.[134]

Action Points

Plastics

- Buy fresh produce at farmers' markets where items are not packaged in plastic.
- Avoid plastics completely for storage and heating of food– switch to glass.
- Get back to the 'good old days' – many cities now have zero waste shops where you can buy in bulk per scoop using your own pre-weighed containers or pack food you buy in glass containers and biodegradable paper bags on site.
- Use glass containers to store drinks and food.
- Use beeswax wrap to store fruit, vegetables and leftover food.
- Use wooden cutting boards over plastic ones.

Cooking

- Replace Teflon pots and pans with stainless steel, ceramic, cast iron or copper.

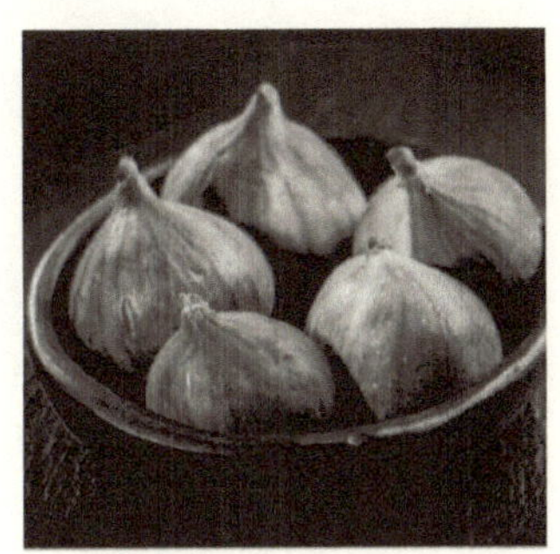

PART FOUR
HEALTH, HEALING
AND HOPE

O you who have believed, eat from the good things which We have provided for you and be grateful to Allah if it is [indeed] Him that you worship. (Quran 2:172)

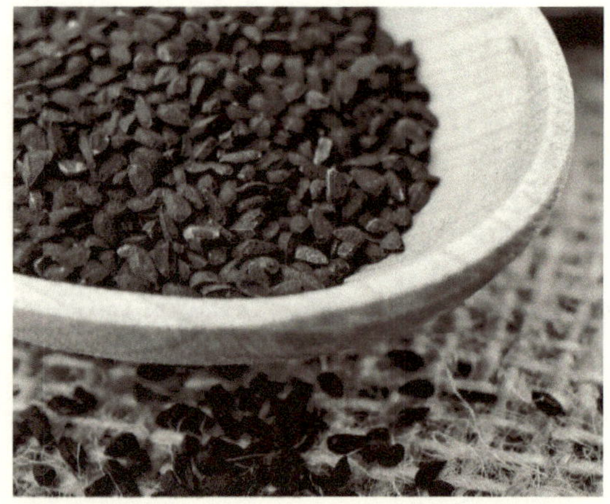

Chapter 23

Total Load: The Sum of the Parts

> **"** *Modern production of foods incorporates a wide range of synthetic chemicals. Many of these chemicals have the potential to be very damaging to humans if they are exposed to high concentrations, or to low concentrations over an extended period of time. (Jeff Gillman, The Truth About Organic Gardening)*[135]

Imagine you're carrying a bag, and then you pick up another one, and another one. At first, you have no problem carrying them; they aren't that heavy after all. Then you load up with another and another and another until, eventually, you are staggering under the weight of everything you're carrying. Your muscles are burning, your fingers are stinging where the bags are pinching your skin, your body aches, you're tired, and you're struggling to take another step. But you keep loading up with more bags until, at last, you can't manage it anymore and buckle under the weight.

This illustrates the concept of 'total load'. The 'bags' are all of the stressors that affect our body and add to what we call our 'total load', a sum of the parts. These stressors can be physical, emotional, chemical, toxic or allergenic, and all add to the total stress load on our bodies.

Allah is all His wisdom has designed our immune system, nervous system and endocrine system in the most incredible fashion, to maintain equilibrium (homeostasis), and our various bodily systems are constantly working very hard towards that ideal balance so as to keep us healthy and functioning. Yet, even our bodies have limits, and, when we keep adding to our total load, what eventually happens is our body reaches a tipping point where the load exceeds the body's ability to cope and maintain balance. Once that happens, tip it will, and symptoms will appear, to let us know we overdid it.

WHAT MAKES UP OUR TOTAL LOAD

FOOD LOADERS

- Allergies (common allergens: dairy, eggs, wheat, chocolate, shellfish, strawberries, citrus, soy, peanuts)
- Food intolerances
- Overeating/excess calories
- Toxins (refined food, pesticides, additives)

GENERAL PHYSICAL LOADERS

- Toxins (environmental and pharmaceutical)
- Sleep deprivation

EMOTIONAL/SPIRITUAL LOADERS

- Stress
- Trauma (Unhealed physical or emotional injuries can potentially impact your immune, hormonal, digestive and neurological systems and can also contribute to weight gain.)
- Depression and anxiety
- Social disconnection
- Spiritual disconnection

CHEMICAL LOADERS

- Environmental chemicals, including pesticides
- Chemicals in the home (cleaning products and body hygiene/ cosmetic products)

Inhalant Loaders
- Pollens, grass, dust, mold, fungi, animal dander, chemicals, pollutants

The Importance of Understanding Total Load

There are many things we may eat that may not harm us as a one-off, or lifestyle choices, like occasional late nights, that we can cope with, but when we continuously add to our load, eventually our bodies will not be able to cope, and we will end up causing ourselves harm.

This applies to what we eat and how much we eat. For example, some food may not be particularly healthy, but our bodies can manage a little – like sugar. Nobody will call sugar a 'health food,' but we can manage with up to about 6 tsp a day according to conventional nutritionists (though I personally would recommend less). Sugar is, after all, a naturally occurring substance, present in most fruits, vegetables, grains and dairy. Problems arise when we continually insist on additional sugar, on top of refined carbs, processed food, additives, excess calories, and a whole host of other food stressors. Our bodies can't handle the overload. We will not feel well and, eventually, we will get sick.

It is not only not smart for us to harm our bodies, it is not permissible, even if we are eating food that is permissible in principle. When we eat continuously or excessively to the point that it causes us harm, we are overstepping the boundaries set by Allah. Scholars have said it is not permissible for anyone to drink so much water or eat so many dates that he will be harmed by them. This applies to other all food and drinks and the combination of these. Shaykh Muhammad ibn Saalih al-'Uthaymeen (may Allah have mercy on him) ruled on this topic:

> *In the case of that which is harmful in conjunction with something else, such as if this food is not compatible with that food, in the sense that if you eat the two foods together it will result in harm, but if you eat them separately that will not result in harm, and the doctor has advised this dietary restriction for one who is sick and has told him, "If you eat it, it will harm you," then it becomes haram (forbidden) for him.*[136]

The Downward Spiral

When we keep adding to our total load, we can end up in a downward spiral. The food we eat puts our body under strain and does not fully nourish us. Stress also affects our energy and hormones. Because we are tired and have less energy, we fuel ourselves on caffeine and sugar and other unhealthy quick fixes to keep going, adding even more to our total load. This affects hormones and stresses our body further, and we end up bouncing between feeling wired and tired, living our days at two extremes. We don't sleep well, so we 'count sheep' on social media, resulting in even less sleep and in lesser quality sleep when we do finally doze off. Feeling ever more tired, we start snapping at those around us, pecking away at the quality of our relationships. Consequently, stress only increases, and we reach for comfort food: more sugar, refined carbs, processed food from familiar brands (the taste of nostalgia), and we add to our total load. And so we go on in a cycle of dis-ease until our body says, 'That's it! I've had enough!' Or, we can decide to stop the downward spiral.

Even before the tipping point, all of those stressors, just like the bags, will weigh us down and affect our lives. We may experience fatigue, moodiness, weight gain, hormonal imbalances, unexplained aches and pains, general lethargy. This, in turn, affects the quality of our lives and our ability to live life to the fullest, to be the best version of ourselves as mother, father, husband, wife, daughter or son – and as a member of our community.

LIGHTENING OUR TOTAL LOAD

Allah has created us with an incredible capacity to cope both physically and mentally, but we have to do our part by following the guidance He has given us as a mercy in the Quran and in the real-life example of His Messenger ﷺ. We need to be careful not to overload our systems. If Allah has promised not to burden us with more than we can bear (Quran 2:286), why do we insistently burden ourselves beyond our threshold?

Do not throw yourselves into destruction. (Quran 2:195)

And do not kill yourselves (nor kill one another). (Quran 4:29)

Allah has given us the guidance we need to maintain health and prevent our total load from reaching a tipping point, and our beautiful deen emphasizes balance in all things. We are encouraged to eat healthy food, avoid excess in all its forms, sleep early, fast and perform the ritual prayer regularly. Human connection and the importance of family and community is continuously emphasized in the Quran and sunnah. We have been given the remedy for stress and worry in the remembrance of Allah, and our success lies in striving for the sake of Allah. These all make up the essential components of good health and gaining greater health; the key is to return to the deen and the guidance of Allah and His Messenger ﷺ, lightening our total load and consciously choosing to nourish ourselves in body, mind and soul for the sake of Allah with the goal of success in this life and the hereafter.

Our lives and choices have become increasingly complex, and some things are harder to avoid than others. Polluted air is tricky to avoid unless we are willing and able to move to a remote countryside destination, but that isn't feasible for everyone. Sometimes finances restrict our options. We can only do what is within our small realm of control to the best of our ability. Alhamdulillah.

Understanding the concept of total load, our personal role in it and its impact on our health means that, by reducing it, we can increase our health and reduce the risk of food and lifestyle-related illness. That realization is half the work, alhamdulillah. Once we know something and understand how our choices are adding up and affecting us, it changes everything, and we can right away start working to reduce it. The key to lightening our total load lies in turning back to the guidance of Allah and His Messenger ﷺ. By improving the quality of the food we eat, the water we drink, avoiding or limiting food which will ultimately add up and harm us, avoiding chemicals that will harm us, getting more sleep and rest and generally prioritizing taking care of ourselves to the best of our ability, we naturally gain health and reduce the risk of disease. We are each a steward of the body with which Allah has blessed us, and we have everything to gain from taking care of it. It is, after all, the only place we have to live.

A Sickened Civilization

With the introduction of commercially processed food and the move away from traditional diets and lifestyles, we have seen a steady global decline in health and a rise in food-related illness. Worldwide, the number of people with diabetes has risen from 108 million in 1980 to 422 million in 2014.[137] Some communities have been hit particularly hard[138] and ethnic low income minorities are among those struggling the most.[139] Native

Hawaiians are some of the world's hardest hit and have high rates of cancer, coronary heart disease and diabetes,[140] having moved away from the traditional diet of their ancestors towards a diet of heavily processed food.

A little closer to home, Muslim communities in the Middle East, Africa and Asia are struggling with serious health issues having moved away from their traditional diets. Muslim countries feature heavily in the top 25 with both the highest rates of obesity and highest rates of diabetes. Our ummah is amongst the sickest in the world. This is because we have moved away from eating food the way Allah made it and the way the Prophet 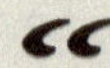 ate it, from following the guidance of the Quran and sunnah in our lives, replacing natural food with the processed food that has crept into our diets and overrun our markets, not realizing that this food has been making us sick.

What an extraordinary achievement for a civilization: to have developed the one diet that reliably makes its people sick! (Michael Pollan, Food Rules: An Eater's Manual [141]

Chapter 24

Gut Health

Digestive problems have reached epidemic proportions globally, with an estimated 30-40% of people complaining about digestive issues.[142] As we have moved away from a natural whole food diet and our lifestyles have changed, our gut health has deteriorated.

Our digestive system is the doorway to the rest of our bodily systems. Every day we swallow food and drinks, supplements and medicines, and our body has the task of figuring out what is friend and what is foe then converting what we eat and drink into usable resources that are delivered to our cells and, finally, neutralizing or getting rid of whatever is harmful or not beneficial. Sounds simple?

Along with your digestive organs that get to work every time you eat, right now, you have about 3-4.5 lbs of bacteria living in your body that help protect you against infections, help run your metabolism and even make vitamins. The estimated 400 to 1,000 or so different species of bacteria in our digestive system are all part of communities that make up your microbiome, and this microbiome largely determines your health.[143]

If the bacterial communities are happy and living in symbiosis (harmony), all is well. When things get out of balance, just as in human communities, bad guys invade and take over, ushering in a wide range of issues, in this case health issues.

Our digestive system does way more than merely break down food so that we can absorb it. As the first line of defense against what we put into our body, it contains about 70% of our immune system. Surprisingly, it is our gut, not our brain, which is responsible for producing the majority of the neurotransmitter serotonin, in your body. In fact, it makes around 80-90% of the serotonin we produce without which we feel depressed. Many other neurotransmitters have also been found in the gut, which is why it is aptly nicknamed 'the second brain'. The gut can also operate solo. Unlike other parts of the body, the digestive system can run on its own even if it is cut off from the brain due to damage to the vagus nerve.[144]

WE ARE WHAT WE EAT

We all know the old adage 'we are what we eat', but it would be more accurate to say that 'we are what we eat, digest, absorb and don't excrete'. The process that our body goes through to ensure our survival is nothing short of miraculous. Subhan Allah.

Ever wondered how an egg turns into energy or muscle in our bodies once we've eaten it? No? Me neither, until I started studying nutrition, but the process is quite astounding. Our bodies cannot actually use food in the form of what we eat. Whether we eat an egg or a bowl of oatmeal, our body can't use either as nutrients or fuel until they have been completely broken down into the tiniest components, and that process takes a whole lot of work.

The process starts automatically every time we eat. While our mouth is chewing and breaking down food mechanically, our saliva, which contains enzymes called amylase, begins to chemically break down carbohydrates, while doing a whole range of other amazing things at the same time. Once in our stomach, the body's blending machine, food is mixed up and broken down further. Parietal cells produce hydrochloric acid (HCl), stronger than battery acid, to aid digestion and also sizzle any pathogens that we may have eaten along with our meal, hopefully neutralizing them. Amazingly, the HCl doesn't burn a hole in our own stomach because the stomach is lined with a protective layer that keeps us safe. The parietal cells also produce intrinsic factor, which allows us to utilize the vitamin B12 in our food. Without this vitamin, we would be susceptible to depression, nervous system issues, muscle weakness, fatigue, and dementia.

Now, cue the sentries! Our gut mucosa is packed with trillions of bacteria and fungi, which are our immune system's first line of defense. Then, there's our lymph system, which enables fat digestion and nutrient absorption and works hard at ferrying fat-soluble nutrients about. It also has the responsibility of initiating immune responses amongst other things.

Once in the small intestine, our food is completely digested and absorbed. A very handy layer of tiny finger-like folds called villi – which are covered by millions of even smaller microvilli, the entire layer being the thickness of just one cell – busy themselves with absorbing nutrients, producing digestive enzymes and blocking any substances that are not beneficial to us from entering our bloodstream. If they lose the ability to tell good from bad, a condition known as intestinal permeability (or leaky gut) in which foreign substances gain access to our bloodstream (the 'world wide web' of our body) and can contribute to a wide range of health conditions. Ensuring our villi and microvilli are in good condition and taken care of is essential to our health.

In connection with our intestines, additional organs play crucial roles. Our pancreas helps to digest food and regulates our blood sugar. Then, there's our liver, which performs over 500 functions, manufactures about 13,000 chemicals and houses 2000 enzyme systems. Among other things, it's responsible for ridding our body of toxins. Also featuring is our gallbladder, which stores the bile our body uses to emulsify fat, and, lastly, our colon absorbs water and remaining nutrients before waste passes out as stool.[145]

All of this is going on every time we eat and for hours afterward. If you haven't thought of it before, now might be a good time to thank Allah for the miracle of your digestive system that is so hard at work to continually keep you nourished and alive. It is food for thought as we realize that what we put into our body will have a direct effect on this entire system.

As with any machine, if there is a malfunction or breakdown in any part of the structure, or if the workers (in this case the colonies of beneficial bacteria that ensure our survival) get killed off or overrun by bad guys, whoever depends on the machine will face serious problems.

DIGESTIVE PROBLEMS CAN BE CAUSED BY SEVERAL THINGS:[46]

- Genetics
- Unhealthy food choices
- Lack of fiber in our diet
- Stress
- Infections
- Environmental toxins
- Prescription medication
- Low hydrochloric acid in our stomach

WHEN THINGS GET OUT OF BALANCE

When our gut microbiome is in in a state of symbiosis, it is in balance. When things get out of balance, we face dysbiosis, which can be expressed by our body in many ways. Research has linked dysbiosis to arthritis, autoimmune disorders, chronic fatigue syndrome, acne, cystitis, eczema, fibromyalgia, food allergies, IBS, restless leg syndrome, and many more conditions. Dysbiosis can be caused by food we eat (or even don't eat), the water we drink, prescription medications, NSAIDS, antacids, proton-pump inhibitors and antibiotics. It can also be caused by other conditions of imbalance such as Heliobacter Pylori, Candida and Small Intestinal Bacterial Overgrowth (SIBO), as well as parasites.[147]

LEAKY GUT (INTESTINAL PERMEABILITY)

Ideally, only beneficial nutrients make it through the tight junctions into our bloodstream, but in the case of intestinal permeability these junctions are compromised, allowing bacterial products, undigested molecules and foreign substances access to otherwise securely-guarded routes. When this happens, the body sets off the alarm bells, activating antibodies, and the body goes into battle mode. This commotion not only causes inflammation of the brush border of the microvilli but can also result in malabsorption of nutrients. Leaky gut is not something with which we are born; it is caused by stress, dysbiosis, household chemicals and contaminants, poor quality food, NSAIDS, birth control drugs, chemo and radiation therapy, and lectins, found mostly in legumes. Lectins in legumes and grains can be reduced by soaking and cooking, sprouting and fermenting them, making the preparation of these nutrient powerhouses key to their status as a health food.[148]

GUT, FOOD AND MOOD: THE GUT-BRAIN CONNECTION

Have you ever found yourself either unable to eat or running for the bathroom when nervous? Feel butterflies in your stomach when excited? Ever had that sinking feeling in your gut when you're about to get 'bad' news? Your gut quite literally has a mind of its own. It's the 'enteric nervous system' that runs our digestive system. It can run even when disconnected from the brain and makes more neurotransmitters than the brain. Just as the way we feel can affect our gut, our gut can affect how we feel. An imbalance originating in the gut can result in behavioral changes; leaky gut has been linked to depression, brain fog, fatigue and poor memory.[149]

STRESS AND DIGESTION

When we are stressed out, our digestive system slows down and can even shut down completely. On the contrary, when we are calm, our digestive system works effectively. If we are in a constant state of stress, like so many of us are, this invariably affects our digestive system. Both stress and emotional upset can play a significant role in many digestive problems as well as in auto-immune issues. Calming down before we eat, eating mindfully, breathing deeply, reciting Quran and starting our meal with du'a and dhikr will all reassure our digestive system that we are ok. Calming our digestive system can have a profound effect not only on our digestion but on our health in general.

THE GUT TAKEAWAY

Understanding just how important our gut is to our overall health is key to our health and wellness. A gut out of balance can lead to malnutrition, inflammation, and chronic illness. It can result in fatigue, lethargy, aches and pains, depression and anxiety, eczema, psoriasis, skin issues and a whole range of other conditions. To take care of our health, we have to take care of our gut and pay extra special attention to the friendly colonies that make up our microbiome.

Heal our gut, and we heal our body. We do this by first avoiding food and other substances that are harmful to our gut, replacing these with health-promoting whole foods and addressing issues like too little HCl or a dearth of digestive enzymes. Food always comes first but sometimes, when we have got our systems so out of balance, there is a need for additional therapeutic intervention. Adding in prebiotics and probiotics, to take care of those friendly colonies, in the form of food is beneficial and supplements may also be used in cases where they are prescribed or recommended by a doctor or healthcare professional. Finally, we can repair our gut through diet and supplements and managing our lifestyle to promote balance and digestive health. What we look forward to when our gut is happy and in balance is not only greater general health but potential reversal of chronic conditions. Working with a doctor or healthcare professional to heal the gut as part of a solution that includes diet, lifestyle and supplement protocols can result in a not just a reduction in symptoms but sometimes remission of conditions entirely.

Chapter 25

The Creator Knows What the Creation Needs

A degree of humility is required when we talk about nutrition, recognizing the limitations of what we currently know and of the science we have and our infinitely limited knowledge and wisdom compared to that of the One who created us.

> *And mankind have not been given of knowledge except a little. (Quran 17:85)*

> *In telling the story of Musa and Al-Khidr, the Messenger of Allah ﷺ said, "And a sparrow came, until it perched on the edge of a boat and pecked at the sea. So Al- Khidr said to Musa, 'My knowledge and your knowledge do not diminish anything from the knowledge of Allah but like what this sparrow diminishes of the sea.'" (Jami Al Tirmidhi)*[150]

Alhamdulillah, we know that Allah created our food to have many incredible healing properties. Black seed is the cure for everything except death,[151] honey is a healing food mentioned in the Quran[152] and the food we eat does not just provide physical benefit but, as in the case of Ajwa dates, can provide spiritual benefits, too.[153]

Most of us eat without giving much thought to the thousands of compounds that make up our daily food. The beautiful colors we see in our fruits, vegetables, and herbs are the result of phytochemicals known as carotenoids and flavonoids. These phytochemicals work in innumerable ways to promote balance in our bodies. To put things into perspective, so far more than 4000 chemically unique flavonoids have been discovered in plants, and we're only just getting started.[154] Flavonoids alone are known to be anti-allergic, anti-carcinogenic, anti-inflammatory, anti-microbial, anti-thrombotic and anti-viral, and they help normalize estrogen, chelate heavy metals and protect our liver, and much remains to be discovered, subhan Allah. Allahu Akbar!

> *And [He has subjected] whatever He multiplied for you on the earth of varying colors. Indeed in that is a sign for a people who remember. (Quran 16:13)*

In the grand scheme of Allah's plan, and with respect to His infinite wisdom, we really don't know a whole lot. We are just scratching the surface with new discoveries, and the more we discover, the more we realize just how infinitely complex nutrition is. In recent years, scientists have found that certain compounds in fruit and vegetables help prevent cancer, but the sheer level of complexity of the chemical makeup of these compounds and how they work synergistically to prevent and cure illness boggles the mind and baffles those studying them.

Alhamdulillah, people have made some crucial discoveries in modern times, some of which have saved lives. A case in point was the discovery that scurvy, a disease that plagued sailors between 1500 and 1800, killing almost 2 million men, was caused by a vitamin C deficiency. Simply dosing sailors with lemon juice would have saved millions.[155] Better yet, shipmates sailing northern seas could have merely swapped their tinned tuna for local fare; more recent studies have shown seal meat to be astoundingly high in vitamin C![156] Science has proved useful, but we don't always get it right, and nutrition science and advice are continuously shifting. Even the simplest 'food pyramid' continues to change shape.

Eggs and avocados were once the nemeses of The Heart Foundation and derided in its food guide; now they are the darlings of the health food industry and rank highly in every health foodie's 'must eat' list. We were told that butter was bad and margarine was good, but it turns out that margarine and trans fats are linked to cardiovascular disease. Oops. We were told that a low-fat diet was the key to health and that sugar could safely replace the tastiness lost with low fat; now we are being told that sugar is the root cause of all our health woes and that fat is our friend. It's no wonder we are all so confused about what is and isn't healthy. Even the experts aren't 100% sure.

What do we do in the midst of all this nutritional 'noise' and ever-shifting diet recommendations? How do we navigate the unpredictably changing tides of science, fancy, fads and food gurus? I believe the most sensible thing any of us can do when it comes to our food is put our trust in the One who made us and made the food we eat because one thing we know for sure is that the Creator knows what His creation needs. He has provided us with abundant food, ecosystems that allow this food to grow and flourish naturally, the rain needed to water the ground, the soil needed for the seeds to germinate and absorb nutrients, the insects needed to pollinate the seeds, and the miracle of seeds themselves and their ability to germinate and grow — each of these things being miracles and signs in themselves. Even in the infertile Arctic, Allah has provided exactly the right balance of nutrients in a form that is edible, and He has blessed us with physical bodies that can digest and utilize nutrients, allowing us, wherever we are in the world, to live, grow, heal and, most importantly, worship Him.

> *It is He who sends down rain from the sky; from it is drink and from it is foliage in which you pasture [animals]. He causes to grow for you thereby the crops, olives, palm trees, grapevines, and from all the fruits. Indeed in that is a sign for a people who give thought. (Quran 16:10–11)*

> *Then eat of what Allah has provided for you [which is] lawful and good. And be grateful for the favor of Allah, if it is [indeed] Him that you worship. (Quran 16:114)*

He has provided us with everything we need, tailor-making our food supply to our seasons and location. Have you ever considered that winter vegetables in higher latitudes are stodgy, higher calorie and help us pad up for the long, cold winter? There is a reason most of us put on extra weight in winter, subhan Allah. In contrast, we see that spring and summer vegetables are lighter and contain more water, ideal for the warmer times of the year. Moreover, tropical climates boast plentiful sweet fruits with high water content, including coconuts that grow abundantly – ideal food for hot and humid weather in which one would sweat a lot and need to stay hydrated. Coconut water is fittingly packed with natural electrolytes which we lose when we sweat. In places like Scandinavia, on the other hand, where warmth and light from the sun are minimal for many months of the year, vitamin D would otherwise be hard to come by, yet Allah, in all His wisdom and mercy, has provided that particular part of the planet with an abundance of fatty fish, one of the best sources of food-based vitamin D. Allah is the Creator and the Provider and He has given us exactly what we need to sustain ourselves in any environment. Of this we have a beautiful example in the lifestyle of the Prophet ﷺ, as it was his custom to eat seasonal and local food.

> *"It was not the custom of the Prophet to restrict himself to one type of food because that is harmful, even if it is the best of food. Instead, he used to eat what was customary among the people of his land.*
>
> *"The Prophet ﷺ used to eat from the fruit of his land when it arrived and this is one of the ways of maintaining good health because Allah, Most Glorified, in His Wisdom, has placed fruits in every land which are a means of preserving the health of its people." (Ibn al Qayyim, Provisions of the Hereafter)*[157]

FOR EVERYTHING THERE IS A SEASON

Eating seasonal, locally grown food is how most cultures have lived for the vast majority of time humans have spent on this planet. When traditional diets prevailed, communities ate whatever was available to them without even knowing what a 'nutrient' was. Natural scarcity also played a role in preventing overconsumption. This has changed dramatically only in the last 70-100 years with the advent of commercial food production and the resultant change in our lifestyle. Correlated with this shift has been the steady and dramatic decline in our health. It seems our cleverness has backfired. Traditional diets fared far better than our modern diet in preventing and limiting disease.

Even in modern times, however, there are a few spots remaining on the planet where, evidently due to diet and lifestyle, the population is largely free of disease. Author Dan Buettner has dubbed these curious communities 'Blue Zones'. One of these zones is a Greek island in the Aegean Sea called Ikaria whose population is remarkably healthy. Ikarians generally live into their 90s, with many centenarians on the island. For the most part, the islanders are unaffected by the diseases the rest of the world is facing, and, amazingly, they mostly remain physically sound and mentally alert right into their old age. Their diets are made up of a diversity of local, seasonal food like fresh fish, vegetables and lots of olive oil, and they get plenty of fresh air, walk a lot, take naps and live as a close-knit community. The interesting thing is that, when islanders move away from Ikaria to other parts of the world, consequently changing their diet and lifestyle, they start getting sick with the same chronic illnesses as everyone else.[158]

The Ikarians aren't alone in living to astoundingly ripe old ages while maintaining mental clarity and vitality. There are several other 'Blue Zones' according to Buettner, where people frequently live to over 100, including Sardinia (Italy), Okinawa (Japan), Loma Linda (California, US) and Costa Rica's isolated Nicoya Peninsula.[159] Common to all of them is a natural whole food diet in harmony with the seasons, reasonable portion sizes, social connection, rest, and exercise – all of these are built into their lives naturally. Their lifestyles are natural, balanced and healthy. Doesn't this sound exactly like the sunnah of the Prophet ﷺ?

It is, in fact, not only sunnah to eat in accordance with the seasons; the Quran specifically advises us to eat from the produce of the earth when it ripens and to not commit excess:

> *And He it is who causes gardens to grow, [both] trellised and untrellised, and palm trees and crops of different [kinds of] food and olives and pomegranates, similar and dissimilar. Eat of [each of] its fruit* **when it yields** *and give its due [zakah] on the day of its harvest. And be not excessive. Indeed, He does not like those who commit excess. And of the grazing livestock are carriers [of burdens] and those [too] small. Eat of what Allah has provided for you and do not follow the footsteps of Satan. Indeed, he is to you a clear enemy. (Quran 6:141-142)*

Jalila Krichi, Holistic Health Coach

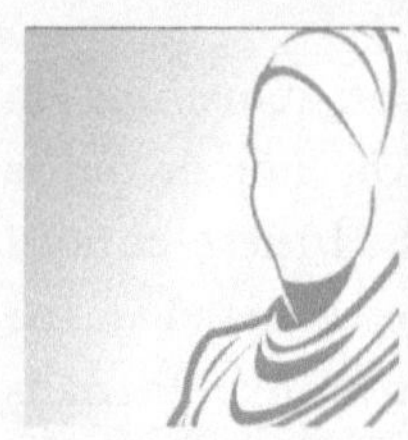

As Muslims, we often take "Islam" to mean submission to Allah SWT through religious rites. As my family and I pursued a more holistic lifestyle to heal ourselves, we realized the wisdom of submitting to Allah SWT's beautiful system of nourishment. Through eating locally grown foods (both animal and vegetable) in their appropriate season, our bodies and minds were able to follow the flow of life through being "grounded" to our environment. Our cravings for detrimental foods abated; our sense of time and flow exempted us from seasonal affective disorder; even the quantities we ate were tempered by the availability in our place of living. We were spared food-decision fatigue, because like a loving mother nourishes her child with the most nutritious and age-appropriate foods, so too does Allah SWT nourish us in season and location. The stress gave way to satiety, our palates found peace and healing took hold.

Yet, not only are we eating more processed food than ever before, we have become accustomed to having every type of food produced anywhere right at our fingertips – all year round and in abundance – without a thought that this food must travel thousands of miles to get to us and be irradiated along the way, dipped in chlorine to maintain freshness or sprayed with chemicals to delay ripening. We have simply come to expect year-round availability as normal and natural.

It is admittedly very enjoyable that we get to taste food from all over the planet without traveling farther than our neighborhood supermarket, and this abundant supply does come with many blessings, alhamdulillah, but having so much available to us has also come with its own set of challenges. In a truly natural environment, we would have a limited supply of food and natural scarcity. If we were growing our food, we would walk out to our garden and choose from whatever was ripe. Anything not ripe we simply wouldn't be eating that night; we'd have to be patient until it was ready to be eaten. Our food would be simple, natural and seasonal. There would be no grumbling at Allah that our avocado wasn't soft yet or that there were no mangoes or fresh lettuce; we'd just accept it with patience, not expecting plants to mature according to our fancy. We would cook based on what was available, not shop based on what we felt like cooking. We would have a deep appreciation of the provision of food and a connection to Allah as the source of that provision. Seasons of scarcity would be times of carefulness. Seasons of harvest would be times of gratitude.

Perpetual global supply means that we no longer have the natural scarcity of seasonal food to limit how much we eat. Even 'healthy' foods are available in abundance, so even being health conscious we may end up overeating because we try to cram all of these foods into our diet. It is easy to eat without realizing that we are overconsuming, eating food upon food upon food. This abundance means that we have to actively limit ourselves to prevent excess consumption and waste, and this can be tough when we are always surrounded by so much from which to choose.

BENEFITS OF EATING SEASONAL LOCAL FOOD

- Food is eaten at its peak freshness.
- Changing repertoire of foods supports the changing needs of the body throughout the year.
- Food positively affects the gut microbiome.
- Appreciation and gratitude increase. We are connected to our food and the One who is providing it.
- Food choices are simplified dramatically, removing the complexity of navigating thousands of imported foods.
- Likelihood of overconsuming even 'healthy food' is reduced.
- Pesticides and irradiation are avoided with locally grown organic food.
- Environmental footprint of our food is reduced.

This is not to say that we should never eat food that isn't seasonal and locally grown, as many other foods can be an immense blessing, but globalization means that it's necessary to be mindful of what we buy and how much we eat, as well as of the environmental footprint of our food. Because we don't have natural scarcity limiting us, we need to be mindful of consuming in excess.

Beyond Chia, Kale and Blueberries

'Healthy' for many of us has come to be associated with certain foods, especially 'super foods'. Chia, kale, blueberries, and quinoa are probably among the first foods that come to mind when we think 'healthy', but the truth is that we don't *need* any of these foods. While these foods are delicious and have wonderful health benefits, as we clearly see from the dietary habits of various traditional cultures, good health does not require an exhaustive variety of imported 'health food' but, rather, simple natural food which Allah has provided in every locale. From the fresh diet of Ikaria's islanders to that of the Okinawans and Sardinians to the food that the Prophet ﷺ himself ate, the lesson is clear: the food Allah has provided may differ by location, but, in all cases – and all places – the foundation of healthy choices is in eating natural whole food, precisely the way Allah made it. If we have the opportunity to include more seasonal and local food in our diet, we stand to reap immense benefits, in shaa Allah. Of course, that does not mean that we never eat food that is not seasonal and local but that, where possible, seasonal and local is a beautiful and healthful choice.

Umm Raqeeb

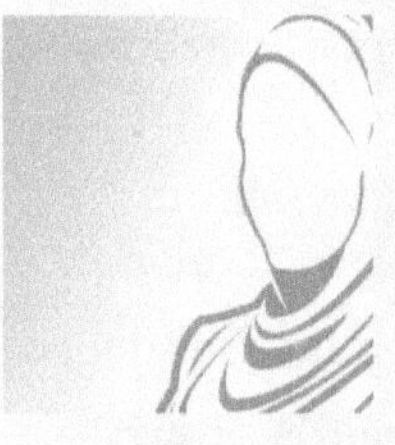

The food scene, at least since I got into it, has been about eating as many colours and textures as possible. The cheffy TV food world is loaded with all this variety... Different types of oils, nutrients from this, that, and foods that we've never even seen before – and you're kind of almost led to believe you're going to die without them. Seriously, I've got to the point where I think, I don't eat blueberries... I must be seriously deficient in blueberryness. And we do that with loads of things because they get hyped up.

Allah's Guidance: Unlawful, Lawful and In Between

Beyond choosing natural whole food as the best option to nourish ourselves, it goes without saying that we also need to be mindful of what Allah has made lawful and unlawful. Allah has prohibited certain foods, not to create hardship for us but for our benefit. Alhamdulillah, avoiding unlawful food is something toward which most Muslims already spend great efforts. More troubling is the seemingly increasing tendency to avoid certain foods as if they are unlawful while Allah has not forbidden them. It is this practice, on the contrary, which is forbidden.

> *O you who have believed, do not prohibit the good things which Allah has made lawful to you and do not transgress. Indeed, Allah does not like transgressors. (Quran 5:87)*

This verse is a sobering reminder to us all. Learned Islamic scholars throughout the ages have trodden with caution to avoid labeling impermissible that which has not been explicitly classified as haram by the Quran and sunnah. Scholars have certainly exercised far more caution on such matters than we often see posted on social media these days.

There are many foods that, when eaten in small quantities and not regularly may be beneficial in principle, or may not cause harm, but these same foods, when consumed daily, continuously, excessively, or in conjunction with other foods, can cause harm. There are also some permissible and even sunnah foods which may be beneficial to some but harmful to others, due to a particular health condition. In such a case as diabetes, dates, dried fruit and honey become harmful substances due to the body's inability to process sugar, which by extension makes them haram for diabetics; it is forbidden in general to knowingly harm one's body. Sheikh al Islam said, "If it is said [by a medical doctor] to a man who has diabetes: Do not eat dates or sweets, then dates and sweets become haraam for him, because they are harmful for him and he has to avoid them, but they are halal for others."[160]

Not transgressing Allah's limits and causing harm to ourselves is what we need to be mindful of when choosing what we eat. If there is any doubt as to the lawfulness of something, it is safer for us to abstain, while avoiding the pitfall of considering something to be unlawful that is not, except in the case of medical advice that bars us from certain foods.

> *'Both legal and illegal things are evident but in between them there are doubtful (suspicious) things, and most of the people have no knowledge about them. So whoever saves himself from these suspicious things saves his religion and his honor. And whoever indulges in these suspicious things is like a shepherd who grazes (his animals) near the Hima*

(private pasture) of someone else and at any moment he is liable to get in it. (O people!) Beware! Every king has a Hima, and the Hima of Allah on the earth is His illegal (forbidden) things. Beware! There is a piece of flesh in the body if it becomes good (reformed) the whole body becomes good but if it gets spoilt the whole body gets spoilt, and that is the heart. (Sahih Bukhari)[161]

We all love to eat what the Prophet ﷺ ate, and we love to eat foods that Allah has mentioned in the Quran, but even with these blessed foods, we have to apply common sense. Not everything is good for everyone. Even blessed sunnah foods and foods mentioned in the Quran might not necessarily be good for you personally. If eating a particular food will cause you harm, that food is not only *not* a health food for you, it is not permissible for you because we are not allowed to harm our bodies. So, for example, if you are lactose intolerant and milk makes you sick, even though Allah mentions milk in the Quran and milk can be a wonderful part of a whole food diet, milk is not a health food for you. If you have diabetes and have been told by doctors to avoid all sugars, then sunnah favorites including honey, dates, dried figs and watermelon, all very high in natural sugar, are not health foods for you. If you have celiac disease, even though the Prophet ﷺ ate wheat, and others can happily eat bread and other gluten grains as part of a natural whole food diet, eating wheat or other gluten-containing grains will make you sick, so these are not health foods for you.

Allah's Infinite Mercy

Even what is specifically impermissible can become permissible when there is an absolute need, under threat of severe injury or death, because it is more important to not harm ourselves.

He has only forbidden to you dead animals, blood, the flesh of swine, and that which has been dedicated to other than Allah. But whoever is forced [by necessity], neither desiring [it] nor transgressing [its limit] - then indeed, Allah is Forgiving and Merciful. (Quran 16:115)

Alhamdulillah, Allah has given us everything we need, natural whole food packed with many healing properties and He has tailor made our provision to suit our environment and our seasonal needs. Out of His mercy, Allah has provided us with a variety of permissible food that not only supports our health and immunity but also tastes amazing and to enjoy and celebrate these foods with gratitude, nourishing our body in the process, can be a beautiful act of worship.

BALANCING BETWEEN PERMISSION AND PLEASURE

Natural food is designed to taste good, yet we do have individual preferences. The Prophet ﷺ had no interest in eating lizard meat[162], but his contemporaries considered it tasty, and he did not forbid them from eating and enjoying it. Personally, I have no taste for fish liver. A number of Muslims prefer not to eat meat at all or avoid animal products altogether. If done out of preference, this is a personal choice that deserves respect. If avoidance is rooted in the belief that meat and other foods are harmful to health and therefore impermissible, it is worth considering that excessive consumption is what is causing harm, not the foods themselves, just as it's excessive production that is harming the earth.

Allah has provided us with every type of food, but man, as we have seen, driven by corporate greed and his desire to boost profits and produce 'more for less', has corrupted our food system and our health.

> *What comes to you of good is from Allah, but what comes to you of evil, [O man], is from yourself. And We have sent you, [O Muhammad], to the people as a messenger, and sufficient is Allah as Witness. (Quran 4:79)*

Chapter 26

Our Bodies Have Been Entrusted to Us and Our Health is a Blessing

This chapter is dedicated to Umm Mansour, without whose support this book would not have been possible. May Allah reward her in this life and the next, and may He shower her and her family with His mercy, ameen.

WE HAVE BEEN CREATED FOR THE SOLE PURPOSE OF WORSHIPPING ALLAH

Life is full of distractions and delusion. Everything is vying for our attention, to do lists are overflowing and most of us exist in a constant state of feeling overwhelmed, just trying to get by. Amidst all this stress, it can be easy to lose sight of what is important. The choices we make each day affect our ability to fulfill our ultimate purpose:

And I did not create the jinn and mankind except to worship Me. (Quran 51: 56)

EVERYTHING HAS A LIMIT, EVEN THE 'GOOD'

Yet, it was not the sunnah of the Prophet ﷺ to stand in prayer non-stop or fast every day of the year. Islam is the religion of balance and moderation, and that applies to everything we do. In that way, everything we do has the potential to fulfill our purpose of worshiping Allah. From fasting in moderation to eating in moderation, striving to achieve balance in all things is a form of worship.

> *Abdullah narrated that Allah's Messenger ﷺ said, "O Abdullah! Have I not been informed that you fast all the day and stand in prayer all night?" I said, "Yes, O Allah's Messenger ﷺ!" He said, "Do not do that! Observe the fast sometimes and also leave them (the fast) at other times; stand up for the prayer at night and also sleep at night. Your body has a right over you, your eyes have a right over you and your wife has a right over you." (Sahih Bukhari)*[163]

If the Messenger of Allah ﷺ prevented his companion from excess in fasting and praying, two of the most beautiful and beneficial acts of worship, because of the rights of his body, his eyes and his spouse, how much more so must this apply to more critical forms of excess in our lives?

OUR BODIES HAVE RIGHTS OVER US

Our body and our health are often the last things we think about – until we get sick and are forced to think about it. There is always so much to do, other people that need help, and, all too often, we put everyone and everything ahead of ourselves. Meeting others' needs is surely important, but eating nourishing food, resting and taking care of ourselves are beautiful acts of worship, too.

If any one of us owned a beautiful property – we'd take care of it. We'd nurture the gardens. We wouldn't let anyone draw on the walls or break furniture. If we had a new vehicle, we wouldn't put soda in the gas tank. But what about our bodies? They are, in fact, both beautiful properties and vehicles. Our bodies are, so to speak, the only place we have to live, and taking care of them is entirely in our best interest, for our time in this world and towards our hopes for the hereafter.

MAINTAINING HEALTH ALLOWS FOR WORSHIP AND IS A FORM OF WORSHIP ITSELF

Our body is a blessing from Allah. Our physical body that holds our spiritual being has been given to us so that we can fulfill our purpose in the life of this world, our ultimate purpose for existence being to worship Allah. It is our body that that allows us to pray, to fast, to love, to work, to eat, to sleep and to care for and serve others. Health is a blessing and a tool for achieving good.

> *Abdullah bin Umar said, "Allah's Messenger 🕌 took hold of my shoulder and said, 'Be in this world as if you were a stranger or a traveler.'" The sub-narrator added: "Ibn Umar used to say, 'If you survive till the evening, do not expect to be alive in the morning, and if you survive till the morning, do not expect to be alive in the evening, and take from your health for your sickness, and (take) from your life for your death.'"* [164]

> *The one among you who wakes up secure in his property, healthy in his body and has his food for the day, it is as if the whole world were brought to him.* [165]

Our bodies are a gift that allows us to worship Allah in this life, and health in body and mind is a blessing that we can use to do good and seek reward from Allah. Yet, neither our bodies nor our health last forever; our bodies are merely on loan to us, and our lives have an expiration date. We belong to Allah, and to Him is our return (Quran 2:156).

All too often, it is only once we lose something, or face the risk of losing something, that we realize and appreciate its value.

> *The Prophet 🕌 said, "There are two blessings which many people lose: (They are) health and free time for doing good." (Sahih Bukhari)* [166]

Even if we have never been seriously sick, smaller reminders generally come each year when we come down with a head cold or the flu. Our head feels full of cotton wool. We ache, we stream, we sniffle and sneeze, we cough, we sweat, we're grumpy and, generally, the most energetic thing we can manage to do is grunt, roll over and put our head under the covers. Our ability to do anything productive dwindles to almost zero.

Fortunately, colds, or even a hefty dose of flu, generally come and go and leave us relatively unscathed. We start to improve after a few days, and, after a week or two, we are back to usual and have completely forgotten the sniffy misery. The low energy, the flat mood, the inability to cope with basic tasks all fade from memory. Most of us probably don't even give it a second thought. We are just happy to be 'back to normal' – doing what we usually do, eating what we usually eat and getting on with life, catching up on our 'to do' list. All is well until we get sick the next time.

> *But if We give him a taste of favor after hardship has touched him,*
> *he will surely say, "Bad times have left me." Indeed, he is exultant*
> *and boastful (Quran 11:10)*

Illness is inevitable. At some point in our lives, however, we are bound to get sick with more than just a cold. Sickness can be a difficult test but also an opportunity for patience and turning to Allah. Sometimes it is only with the sharp reminder of severe illness that we realize that the blessings of health and time as tools for doing good; while often plentiful, they are finite resources.

> *And We will surely test you with something of fear and hunger*
> *and a loss of wealth and lives and fruits, but give good tidings to*
> *the patient. (Quran 2:155)*

As anyone who has lost their health knows, the pain of sickness is not only in the illness itself but in the slipping away of the abilities they once had. The ability to make sujood. The ability to fast in Ramadan. The energy to spend time with their kids without being exhausted and in agonizing pain. The ability to walk or see, having lost their legs or their sight to diabetes. The ability to eat and enjoy the taste of food rather than receive liquid nutrition through a tube. Their patience with Allah's decree stands to gain reward, yet their hearts ache to regain what they had before, their hearts miss the feeling of the cold floor on their forehead in prostration to their Lord, their hearts yearn to be able to join in fasting the month of Ramadan.

If we are not already in compromised health, the only thing standing between it and us is time. Before that happens, we have an opportunity each day to use whatever health we have to seek Allah's pleasure. What we have today we may not have tomorrow, and the choices we make today will affect our tomorrow, our next week, our next month, our next year and our hereafter.

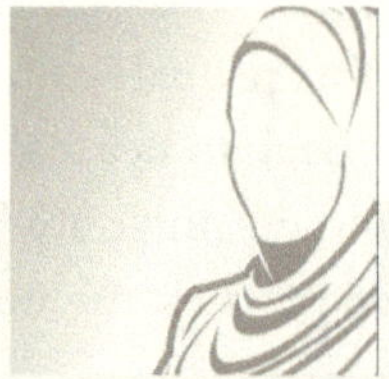

Um Haleema

Complications in digestive health come with its many consequences. One of these was the heart ache of not being able to fast during the blessed month of Ramadan. Despite the sadness and sense of loss I felt not being able to participate during this time, I always understood and believed that there was just as much barakah in this month for me as there was for anyone else. I could still worship Allah and gain rewards in numerous different ways. I could facilitate suhoor and iftar for my family, for the needy, perform extra prayers and purify my heart and intentions to please Allah SWT. We have to remember in essence Ramadan is a training ground where we learn self-control, mercy and worthy moral behaviours so that we are able to make this our way of living. Abstaining from food is not the only form of worship practiced during this month. We try a little harder to rehearse these traits in order to ingrain these into our habitual daily lives, and there is a form of worship available to everyone regardless of their conditions.

During the last decade or so I have been on a most incredible journey. A journey of realisation, re-discovery and resolution. Realising that Allah SWT is the One who is in charge, and there is only so much I have control over. Re-discovering the aspects of my life that I could refine and develop in order to enhance my wellbeing. This soon led me to make firm resolutions to inculcate change in my diet, physical and emotional health and mental stability. It's astounding what the combination of will-power and dua can do. Change was slow and gradual, with many peaks and lows but I was moving in the right direction Alhamdulillah. A decade on from that very first heart ache I quietly celebrated a full month of fasting by whispering a prayer of gratitude to my Lord. I am truly in awe of my Lord and of the journey He granted me.

Chelsea, Wellness Muslimah

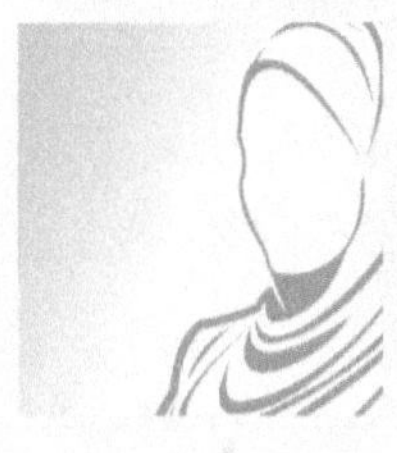

After I was diagnosed with PCOS in 2016, my health priorities changed. Food was no longer my enemy. It was no longer something I had to fear would make me "fat." Instead, food became my medicine. It became a healing. Allah has blessed us with so many beneficial foods that provide us energy, nourishment, strength. After switching to a more natural, whole-foods based diet, I was able to, by the will of Allah, regulate my cycles and improve my PCOS symptoms. Nutrition has been, and always will be, my first step towards living a healing lifestyle, alhamdulillah.

Sister Carol

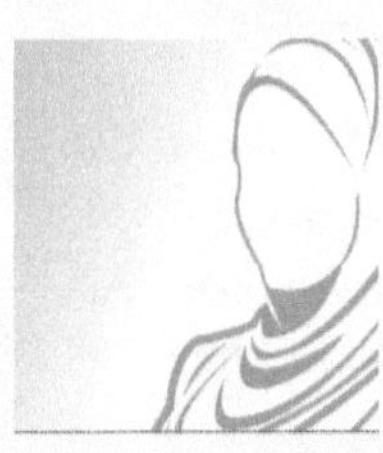

When I developed Polymyalgia Rheumatica at age 53, I knew my world was going to change. Suddenly my energetic and healthy self couldn't move. I found myself on medication that created more problems than it solved and chronic joint pain and stiffness was probably going to be a fact of life for the foreseeable future. I determined I was going to beat it by adapting my diet.

WE HAVE BEEN GIVEN CLEAR GUIDANCE

Allah has created our bodies as beautiful and complex machines with hundreds of thousands of processes taking place every minute. Who knows better what the creation needs than the Creator Himself? He has not left us to wander blindly and figure things out for ourselves. The body of knowledge humans share has not been discovered randomly. Numerous prophets and messengers have relayed critical guidance since the beginning of humanity. Today, we find all the guidance we need to live a healthy and balanced life compiled in the Quran and sunnah. We have been guided on how to eat, how we sleep, how to manage stress and how to prioritize in line with our ultimate purpose. Alhamdulillah, the remedy for all of our stress, our excess and our dwindling health lies in the guidance provided by the One who created us. We trust the Prophet ﷺ set the best example in all areas of living, so to emulate his example is the recipe for success in both this life and the hereafter.

> *And obey Allah and obey the Messenger and beware. And, if you turn away — then know that upon Our Messenger is only [the responsibility for] clear notification. (Quran 5: 92)*

We are stewards of our body, and every day we have an opportunity to take care of the body with which Allah has blessed us, alhamdulillah, by following the guidance He has given us. While children learn to look after their belongings and gifts they receive, we, too, have much still to learn from our Creator to look after the gift of our bodily health.

> *Indeed the first of what will be asked about on the Day of Judgment — meaning the slave (of Allah) being questioned about the favors — is that it will be said to him: "Did We not make your body, health, and give you of cool water to drink?" (Tirmidhi)[167]*

> *The son of Adam will not pass away from Allah until he is asked about five things: how he lived his life, how he utilized his youth, with what means did he earn his wealth, how did he spend his wealth, and what did he do with his knowledge. (Tirmidhi)[168]*

We are not passive participants in our health journey, biding our time and waiting for the inevitable. Our choices directly affect our health and wellbeing, and we will be questioned about them. After a lifetime (or even a mere childhood) of indulging in a massive amount of sugar, refined carbohydrates, and other unhealthy food, we can only be as surprised about Type 2 Diabetes as we'd be about a bruised finger after hitting it with a hammer. Neither should we be surprised that we are targeted by sly marketing techniques in connection with something as necessary to our survival as food, as we have been warned of this. The shaitan is ever a deceiver, aiming high and low to lead us astray.

> *[Satan] said, "Because You have put me in error, I will surely sit in wait for them on Your straight path. Then I will come to them from before them and from behind them and on their right and on their left, and You will not find most of them grateful [to You]." (Quran 7:16-17)*

> *"And I will mislead them, and I will arouse in them [sinful] desires, and I will command them so they will slit the ears of cattle, and I will command them so they will change the creation of Allah." And whoever takes Satan as an ally instead of Allah has certainly sustained a clear loss. (Quran 14:119)*

Being duped by shaitan's evil ways is a tragic way to lose our health, while taking care of our body – physically, mentally, emotionally and spirituality – is a beautiful way to worship Allah. Not only do we feel better, we are able to be better versions of ourselves – for ourselves, for our loved ones and for Allah.

THE HEALTH YOUR GAIN FROM MAKING GOOD CHOICES YOU CAN USE TO DO GOOD

Just as we can put the savings we gain from purchasing less food overall towards higher quality, if more expensive, food, we can put the health we gain from making good choices towards good or better deeds.

> *The Messenger of Allah said, "Make the most of five things before five others: life before death, health before sickness, free time before becoming busy, youth before old age, and wealth before poverty." (Saheeh al-Jaami')*[169]

FOOD AFFECTS MORE THAN JUST PHYSICAL HEALTH

The food we eat affects us not only physically but emotionally, mentally and spiritually as well. Aside from the haram, which most Muslims already avoid, empty calories and greasy, sugary, refined food that doesn't contain any nourishment can negatively affect us, sapping our energy, affecting our mood, our sleep, our choices and our desire to engage in that which benefits us. When we eat this sort of food, we are far more likely to want to flop on the couch and stare at a screen than go for a walk, read Quran or pick up a book that increases us in beneficial knowledge.

When we eat unhealthy food, we don't feel like getting up for fajr or praying tahajjud. By choosing to eat food that nourishes us, we not only take care of our body physically, but we increase our ability to do that which benefits us and leave that which is excessive, harmful or not beneficial.

Not only does the type of food we eat affect us but the amount we eat affects us. Overeating food is among the four poisons of the spiritual heart identified in <u>Purification of the Soul</u>.[170]

FOUR POISONS OF THE HEART

1. Unnecessary talking
2. Unrestrained glances
3. **Too much food**
4. Keeping bad company

Sister Khalida

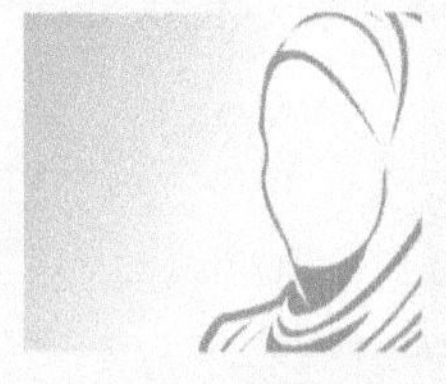

It took me a long time to realize that eating a bowl of potato chips, especially at night, would affect not only my mood, sleep, and choices at my next meal but also that eating junky foods like chips actually affected my desire to read and learn. When I eat junk, I am much more likely to "veg-out" and watch Netflix rather than finish the Autobiography of Malcolm X, for example, or involve myself in something that is beneficial to my life. In short, the way I choose to eat has a lasting effect on the choices I make in the short term and the long term because choices made in the short term become habits that affect my life in the long term.

TRAINING OURSELVES

It is not always easy to say no to our desire to eat whatever we want, but, by striving to do this, we train ourselves to say no to our desires when they clash with what is reasonable or appropriate, and we are able to overcome them. As Ibn al Qayyim explained, "Whoever gives up striving completely, his religious motives will become weak, and his motive to follow his desires will become strong, but when he trains himself to go against his desires, he can defeat them whenever he wants."[171] He also said in relation to striving, "The believer who is striving knows that goodness will remain and will prevail, no matter how intense the darkness, how great the calamity, how prevalent and widespread the evil and how many limits are transgressed. And Allah is the One Whose help we seek."[172] A healthy diet indeed involves training and disciplining oneself to observe reasonable limits, and it must start with the spiritual heart.

DOING OUR PART - TYING OUR CAMEL TO A TREE

None of us want to get sick. Nobody wants to make choices that make them sick. Nobody wants to make choices that will make their family sick. Alhamdulillah, we are not burdened by Allah with more than we can manage and Allah does not wish to cause us hardship. We are only asked to do what is reasonably within our control. We lock our car, for example, in an attempt to prevent theft but don't erect meteorite shields every time we park it in the open. In an exemplary lesson recorded in hadith, the Prophet ﷺ instructed a man about to enter the mosque, who had considered leaving his camel in Allah's care while he prayed, to "tie [his] camel to a tree and *then* trust in Allah."[173]

The challenge we face in our modern times is knowing how to choose a tree that is wholesome and strong rather than one weakened by inner rot. We face the task of distinguishing which ordinary items are rotten from deception, having to navigate deceit on an industrial scale in the form of insincere marketing and advertising by corporations. We are living in one of the most challenging times in food history, surrounded by more food than ever that is designed to look better and taste better even if it makes us feel worse. We can only do our best to select trustworthy 'trees' in securing and maintaining what is valuable to us, including our health. When we succeed, by making good choices and by the grace of Allah, in nourishing ourselves, physically, mentally and spiritually, we can be a better version of ourselves, be a greater benefit to those around us and better worship Allah.

Khadija Abdus Sabur, Woman by Nature

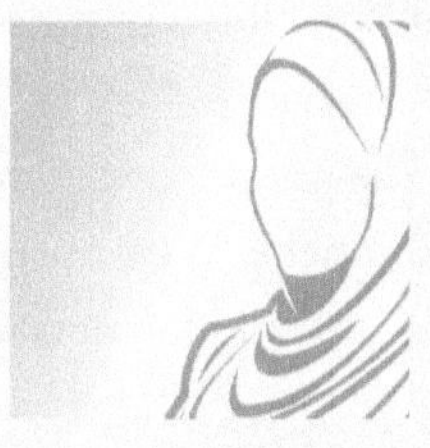

Health is a holistic experience. If we don't get adequate sleep, we often eat poorly in an attempt to get through the day. If we eat poorly, we can experience brain fog and sluggishness that impedes our effectiveness at work and school. If we're then experiencing cognitive issues, we're less likely to display patience and understanding, leading to strained relationships. Your health is your biggest asset and it's all connected.

Chapter 27

How the Prophet ﷺ Ate

This chapter is dedicated to Um Yusef, without whose care, diligence, patience, attention to detail and accuracy and valuable input this book would not be what it is today. May Allah grant her and her family the highest station in Jannah, ameen.

We all want to know what exactly the Prophet ﷺ ate? How much did he eat? When did he eat? How many times a day did he eat? When I face these questions, to much disappointment, I cannot give a definitive answer on detailed specifics of every aspect of the Prophet's ﷺ diet. While we do know many of the foods that the Prophet ﷺ loved to eat, we do not find recorded comprehensive details of *exactly* what he ate every day, what time he ate, exactly how much he ate at every meal, how many meals he ate every day or what ratio of fats, proteins and carbohydrates he ate.

What we have been given rather are guidelines, a framework for a style of eating that is appropriate to our physical design and pleasing to our Creator. Alhamdulillah, the lack of specificity is a great mercy as it accommodates the natural variance between people. We are all different and have different needs and constitutions and circumstances. Within the guidelines there is space for personal preferences and individual needs, budgets and differences in local availability.

I believe there is great wisdom in not only the beautiful example we have to follow but also in the flexibility that these guidelines allow. The lack of specificity naturally accommodates the immense variance between people, places, preferences, individual needs and local availability. We are all so different: a pregnant mother looking after a troop of children does not have the same dietary needs as someone who is sedentary and has a sluggish metabolism. A worker manually tilling a field in India for 14 hours a day needs a whole lot more calories than someone spending those same 14 hours behind a computer in a high rise. A growing teenager needs more food than a small child. Someone recovering from surgery or with a chronic illness may have specific nutritional needs and perhaps food restrictions different from someone in optimum health. A health food for one may not be a health food for another. Even within our personal constitutions, we are all different. Some of us may do better with higher fat diets, others thrive on carbs. Some of us may like a certain food but not be so fond of another. We are all different.

In spite of our differences, however, the *foundations* of a healthy diet remain the same for everyone and because our food system has been so severely compromised, it has become essential for us to actively choose food that is natural and wholesome specific to our individual needs. In making the best possible choices we can with the resources we have and striving to eat food the way Allah made it and the way the Prophet ﷺ ate it, we seek Allah's pleasure and reward including that of health and wellness in this life. The beauty of the guidance we have is that it gives us clear guidelines on how to eat while also being flexible, accommodating individual and environmental differences and comprising the incredible abundance and variety of food that Allah has provided in every habitable place in the world.

Khadija Abdus Sabur, Woman by Nature

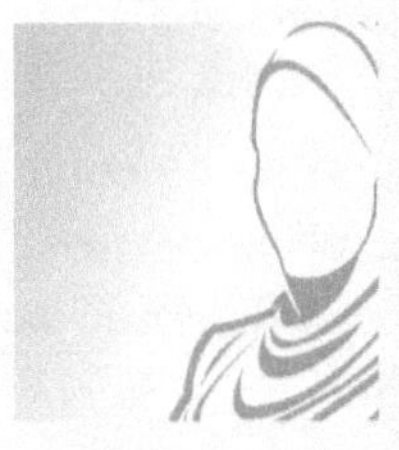

So much of what we're taught about health and eating is far removed from our fitra and the prophetic example. However, by choosing to embrace a more divine way of eating – we can literally change the makeup of our bodies. Adopting a natural diet greatly contributed to my overcoming a debilitating case of lupus back in 2004, by Allah's permission – and I've seen it contribute to greater health and longevity for many others as well.

NATURAL WHOLE FOOD

As a starting point, the Prophet ﷺ ate natural whole food. If we let our minds wander back in time to imagine Medina's market as it was in his time, it's a far cry from our jump forward in time to MacDonald's arches in every city worldwide, fast food outlets at every turn, food delivery services, drive-thru lines for everything from full meals to coffee, online food shopping and countless supermarkets and corner stores all stocked to the brim with food, food, and more food.

Or should we call it 'food'? While we are constantly bombarded with variety like never before, much of what is available is neither nutritious nor healthy. In contrast, food in the time of the Prophet ﷺ would have been 100% natural with nutrients intact: wholesome food exactly the way Allah made it. There would have been no need for organic labeling because ALL food was organic. In the time of the Prophet ﷺ, people did not agonize over the nutrient content of food or need to spend hours poring over labels to decode fat and sugar content, what is and isn't GM, what is artificial and what is 'natural', what the listed additives all do and whether they are safe. They did not have to worry about pesticides or genetic modification because agriculture was yet uncorrupted. Honey, so loved by the Prophet ﷺ and honored in the Quran, would have been natural, raw and pure. The Prophet ﷺ would not have had to wonder if it had been made by bees exposed to sugar water, if it was contaminated with pesticides or if it had been irradiated to the point of losing its healing properties. Meat would have been naturally produced, free of antibiotics and growth hormones and animals would have been pasture-raised. Wholegrains would have been used to make the staple bread of the time, not refined flours stripped of nutrients. In a nutshell, food was exactly the way Allah made it. Natural, wholesome and pure.

Food being natural, the Prophet ﷺ wouldn't have known the year-round availability of food to which we are accustomed today. Food would have been grown and eaten according to the seasons, and people would have eaten whatever was available at the marketplace or from family farms. Availability of fresh produce would have been determined by whatever was ripe from among whatever could naturally grow in the oases of Medina. There were no fridges or freezers, no commercial mass processing, no artificial additives or preservatives. Just seasonal, organic, locally-grown food supplemented by occasional 'imports' brought in by trading caravans from as far away as Syria and Yemen. Food would have been 'processed' in homes in basic, sustainable ways without the use of harmful or suspicious chemicals: drying, preserving with salt or vinegar, stone-grinding, fermenting.

To be able to supplement seasonal and local food supplies with import from neighboring regions was a great blessing in the time of the Prophet ﷺ as it is today, especially in seasons of natural scarcity like long cold winters and in places where crops did not yield sufficiently, perhaps due to drought or flooding. No longer do we have to prepare for the long winter months by storing, drying and canning food at home or fear starving if we did not have a good yield. There are certainly some benefits, including convenience and constant availability, in the ability to transport and store food on such a global scale but globalization and commercial food production have sparked a whole new set of food challenges. To eat natural whole food as it was in the time of the Prophet ﷺ now takes a degree of effort. Even to identify what truly constitutes natural whole food takes effort. Such a task is no longer ordinary. Commercialization of food has made simple, healthy choices a trial; to eat natural whole food the way it was consumed in the time of the Prophet ﷺ requires knowledge and conscious food selection. Understanding the nature of food in the time of the Prophet ﷺ and how our food system has been compromised has become essential for knowing how to make the best choices.

A fundamental principle of our deen is that we should do our bodies no harm. Because our food system has been so corrupted, to avoid causing harm to our bodies, we can no longer just buy whatever is available in the market. We need to know where our food is coming from and what is in it so that we can make the best possible choices and eat food as close as possible to the way Allah made it and to the way the Prophet ﷺ would have eaten it.

Ibn al-Qayyim (may Allah have mercy on him) summed up for us the practice and the teachings of the Prophet ﷺ with regard to food and drink, which he derived from authentic ahadith:

"The practice of the Prophet ﷺ was not to reject what was available, and not to go out of his way to seek that which was not available. No good food was brought to him but he ate it unless he had no

appetite for it, in which case he left it but did not forbid it. He never criticized any food. If he wanted it, he ate it; otherwise, he would leave it. The Prophet ﷺ refrained from eating lizard meat because he was not used to it, but he did not forbid it to the ummah. He ate sweets and honey, which he liked. He ate camel meat, mutton, chicken, bustard, onager, rabbit, and seafood. He ate grilled meat and both fresh and dry dates... He did not refuse good food, and he did not go out of his way to seek it; instead, he would eat what was available, but if it were not available he would be patient, and he would tie a stone to his stomach because of hunger. Three new moons in a row would be sighted, and no cooking fire would be lit in his house." [174]

The Prophet ﷺ ate any good food that he encountered, but certain gems stand out as particularly blessed as they are associated with not only nourishment but healing as well. If you don't already include these in your diet, do consider adding them!

VINEGAR

The Prophet ﷺ praised vinegar[175] as a condiment, and there are immense health benefits to including natural vinegar in our diet. Natural, raw organic vinegar that has not been filtered is packed with health benefits. Drinking 1 Tbsp of raw organic vinegar (widely available today) in 8 oz of tepid water first thing in the morning can have immense benefits for gut health. The same mix before meals can also help aid digestion. Vinegar can also be used in salad dressings, marinades and cooking and as a condiment by itself.

BLACK SEED

The Prophet ﷺ associated black seed with healing "everything except death."[176] You can chew a pinch-worth along with a teaspoon of honey, add it to food and even make tea from it.

OLIVE OIL

Loved and recommended by the Prophet ﷺ for both use on food and application to our skin,[177] olive oil is one of the most heart-healthy foods we can eat. Use high quality, cold pressed olive oil daily and drizzle it on food such as salads. You can also use olive oil to sauté food.

Honey

Use raw, organic, unpasteurized honey as a blessed healing food[178] – try to find a safe and recommended source of local honey. Less is more – it is better to eat a lesser quantity of excellent quality honey than more of a 'honey' that is not beneficial. 1 portion = 1 tsp (not 3 Tbsp in your morning porridge).

Dates

Dates are mentioned in both the Quran and sunnah, with special mention made of Ajwa dates. If you have them available to you, then alhamdulillah. Try to eat seven each day.

> *I heard Allah's Messenger ﷺ saying, "Whoever takes seven Ajwa dates in the morning will not be affected by [black] magic or poison on that day." (Sahih Bukhari)*[179]

For a comprehensive list of sunnah foods as well as traditional medicine used in the time of the Prophet ﷺ, consult Ibn Al Qayyim's *Medicine of the Prophet*.

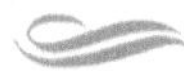

The Sunnah of Eating

Beyond all the information about *what* the Prophet ﷺ ate, there are many more narrations about *how* he ﷺ ate. The more we can follow his example, the greater the reward and the greater the benefit for us in this life and the hereafter, in shaa Allah. Many we may already know, and many we may already be implementing, but reminders always benefit the believers, so following is a list of authentic ways of the Prophet ﷺ related to eating, drinking and fasting.

The Prophet ﷺ instructed us to mention Allah, eat with the right hand and eat what is nearest us.

> *"Mention Allah's Name (i.e., say 'bismillah' before starting to eat), eat with your right hand, and eat from what is near you." (Sahih Bukhari and Sahih Muslim)*[180]

The Prophet ﷺ recommended and practiced eating small portions.

> *"The human does not fill any container worse than his stomach. It is sufficient for the son of Adam to eat what will support his back. If this is not possible, then a third for food, a third for drink and a third for his breath." (Jami at-Tirmidhi)*[181]

The Prophet ﷺ said food for one can suffice for two, et cetera.

> *"Food for one (person) suffices two, and food for two (persons) suffices four persons and food for four persons suffices eight persons." (Sahih Muslim)*[182]

The Prophet ﷺ ate with three fingers which he licked clean after eating.

> *The Messenger of Allah ﷺ used to eat (food) with three fingers and he licked his hand before wiping it. (Sahih Muslim)*[183]

The Prophet ﷺ had preferences and loved sweet flavors and honey.

> *Allah's Messenger ﷺ used to love sweet edible things and honey. (Sahih Bukhari)*[184]

The Prophet ﷺ drank water in three gulps.

> *Anas reported that Allah's Messenger ﷺ used to breathe three times in the course of a drink (i. e. he drank in three gulps). (Sahih Muslim)*[185]

The Prophet ﷺ chose not to eat food unfamiliar to the land of his people, but he did not prohibit others from eating it.

> *A roasted mastigure (lizard) was brought to the Prophet ﷺ who stretched his hand towards it to eat it. But it was said to him, 'It is a mastigure.' So he withdrew his hand. Khalid asked, 'Is it unlawful to eat?' The Prophet ﷺ said, 'No, but it is not found in the land of my people, and that is why I do not like eating it.' So Khalid started eating (it) while Allah's Messenger ﷺ was looking at him. (Sunan Nasaa'i)*[186]

The Prophet ﷺ recommended eating with others.

Some of the companions of Messenger of Allah ﷺ said, "We eat but are not satisfied." He ﷺ said, "Perhaps you eat separately." The companions replied in the affirmative. He then said, "Eat together and mention the name of Allah over your food. It will be blessed for you." (Abu Dawud)[187]

The Prophet ﷺ did not eat reclining.

"I do not eat reclining (against a pillow)." (Sahih Bukhari)[188]

The Prophet ﷺ did not criticize food.

The Prophet ﷺ never criticized any food (he was invited to) but he used to eat if he liked the food, and leave it if he disliked it. (Sahih Bukhari) [189]

The Prophet ﷺ cleaned then ate food that was accidentally dropped.

"When anyone of you drops a mouthful, he should remove anything filthy from it and then eat it, and should not leave it for the Satan." (Sahih Muslim)[190]

The Prophet ﷺ did not leave food in his dish.

He also commanded us that we should wipe the dish saying, "You do not know in what portion of your food the blessing lies." (Sahih Muslim)[191]

The Prophet ﷺ made du'a for hosts who had provided him with a meal.

"O Allah, bless them in what You have provided them as a sustenance and forgive them and have mercy upon them." (Sahih Muslim)[192]

The Prophet ﷺ used to fast Mondays and Thursdays.

The Messenger of Allah ﷺ used to observe a fast on Mondays and Thursdays. (At-Tirmidhi)[193]

The Prophet ﷺ recommended fasting the days of the three full-moon nights each month.

> *"The Messenger of Allah ﷺ used to command us to fast the days of the white (nights): thirteenth, fourteenth and fifteenth of the month. He said, 'This is like keeping perpetual fast.'" (Sunan Abi Dawud, Sahih Al-Albani)[194]*

The Prophet ﷺ recommended we eat suhur prior to a day of fasting.

> *"Take suhur as there is a blessing in it." (Sahih Bukhari)[195]*

The Prophet ﷺ recommended that we hasten to break the fast once the sun has set.

> *"The people will remain on the right path as long as they hasten the breaking of the fast." (Sahih Bukhari)[196]*

The Prophet ﷺ recommended fasting 3 days a month

> *"O Abdullah bin Amr, you fast all the time and you do stand (in prayer) at night, but if you do that your eyes will become sunken and you will become exhausted. There is no fast for one who fasts every day of his life. Fasting a lifetime means fasting three days each month." (Sunan an-Nasa'i)[197]*

Unlocking the Benefits of the Sunnah with the Key to Healthy Eating

Increasing good habits inspired by the sunnah has a very rewarding effect, but trying to remember and apply all of the sunnah at once can feel overwhelming. As part of our step by step approach, we aim to make small, regular and consistent additions to our lives, which is sunnah in itself, always focusing on seeking Allah's help and His pleasure in this life and the hereafter.

Of course, every sunnah of the Prophet ﷺ has immense benefit. For the purpose of trying to make better choices regarding food and its effect on the body, however, I have consolidated food-related advice from the sunnah into three categories, represented by three teeth on a key, the **Key to Healthy Eating**. Fittingly, the teeth are echoed by Michael Pollan's advice in *Food Rules: An Eater's Manual,* in which he offers the key to healthy eating in just 7 words, "Eat food. Not too much. Mostly plants." When I was looking at the diet of the Prophet ﷺ and the example of how he ﷺ ate, comparing it to our modern diets, I could see that there is one overall principle that encompasses entirely the multiple ways in which we have gone wrong and what we need to do to get back on track. Each prong of this visual aid is related to details in the sunnah which describe how the Prophet ﷺ ate. They involve, in respective order, how we eat, how much we eat and how often we eat.

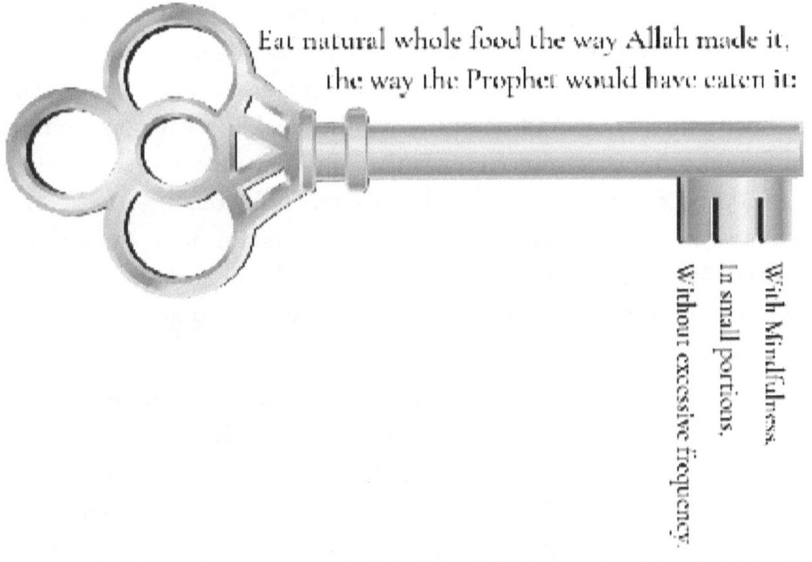

With Mindfulness

Chances are you already say 'bismillah' before eating, and, if you have children, you have taught them to do the same. While most of us probably remember to say bismillah before we tuck into a meal, we might be saying it more out of habit than anything else, with our minds a million miles away – thinking about 'to do' lists, worrying or planning for what's next or maybe scrolling through Facebook or Instagram or posting a snap of our meal.

Changing our level of consciousness when we say bismillah at the start of a meal can have a profound effect on us. Saying bismillah with sincerity and mindfulness, really thinking about what you are saying, requires slowing down, quieting down and being present in the moment. It can be useful to consider the bismillah as a sort of moment of silence, even if pronounced aloud. Consider the effect of taking a moment at the start of eating to be mindful of the food you are eating and of the One who has provided it for you, as well as of anyone who has had a hand in it before it reached your plate: those who grew it, harvested, transported, purchased, prepared, served. It's a rare case that we do all of those jobs ourselves. It prevents us from eating mindlessly, helps improve our choices and helps prevent overeating. It is also beneficial, at the moment of the bismillah, to consider those with whom you are sharing the meal – and those with whom you are not sharing the meal, those in your home or your neighborhood or your city, whether they have food to eat or might have no meal at all. According to hadith, our individual portion – even a sunnah-sized individual portion – could be enough to share with one other person; we can't feed the entire world with one dish, but we can at least consider those in our vicinity when we lift our fingers or fork and say bismillah.

The simple act of *consciously* saying 'bismillah' can bring us into the moment and can help us appreciate what we have and cultivate gratitude. It can help remind us of the blessings and favor of our Lord and remind us of our purpose and why we need to nourish our body. Such reminders are in themselves rewarding. But there's more: slowing down and being mindful also helps with digestion. It causes our bodily systems to shift from a sympathetic state, in which we are ready for action and in 'fight or flight' mode (in which digestion is actually inhibited) to a parasympathetic state, in which the body calms down and more energy can be directed toward the gut, enhancing digestion. Chewing thoroughly further supports the digestion process, and eating slowly allows time for the gut to let the brain know when you've had what it can handle.

Mindfulness at mealtimes can also help to limit what types of food we eat. Beginning with bismillah and asking Allah to bless the food you're about to eat may feel awkward if what you're about to eat is a huge slice of cake dressed in sugar paste and layered with buttercream. Seriously? Bless the sugar paste and buttercream? In that case, eating is much easier with your mind switched off! In fact, much commercially processed and convenience food falls into this category, and, unless we're reading labels carefully, we may have no idea how much sugar we're consuming, even by way of savory foods, or how much salt or synthetic ingredients. Instead of buying lots of processed food and keeping ready-made snacks and sweets in the house, we can support food-related mindfulness by making what we eat and eating what we make. If we want to eat cake, we can make it from scratch with trusted basic ingredients rather than buying it or using a ready-mix. As we pour multiple cups of sugar into a bowl and cut in a large lump of butter, we begin to realize all that goes into cake baking. Being mindful of the process and the effort and ingredients involved is likely to make us think twice the next time we want to eat cake, or at least the next time we are tempted to purchase commercially-produced cake.

As You Say 'Bismillah'

- **Think about the blessing of the food you have, the food that Allah has provided from His bounty.** The greatest blessing in food is its nutrient content by which we are nourished and truly satisfied. Remember the thousands of brothers and sisters around the world who are going hungry or who eat 'food' but are not nourished, and be grateful for the food you have. I feel especially grateful since seeing an interview of a young Arab boy living in a war zone. When asked what he would love to eat, he replied, "Cucumbers." Not candy, not cake, not chips, not pizza. All he wanted was fresh cucumbers. And it's not only those in impoverished war zones who crave fresh, nutritious food:

Umm Yusef

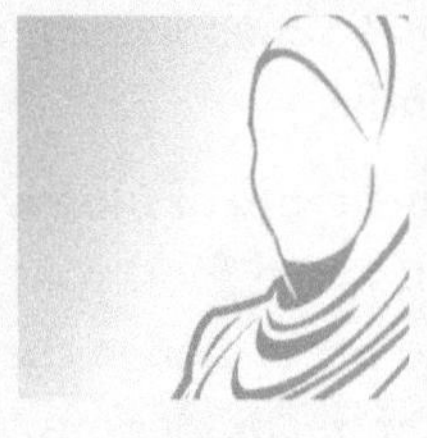

I was taken aback when I discovered my son had, on more than one occasion, agreed to sell his daily carrot, which I packed in his school lunch, to a classmate who always brought plenty of money to school only to find the same boring options day in and day out at the canteen: white bread with a bit of cheese or white bread with a bit of za'atar. All the boy wanted was some nutrition, and he was willing to offer a hefty sum. I'm ashamed to say my son collected ten dirhams (almost three dollars) per carrot! I'm even more ashamed to say he used the money to buy white bread with cheese!

- **Connect with your food, think about where it came from and give thanks.** Think about the earthly source of your meal. When you eat meat, consider the animal that surrendered its life and give thanks. Think about the vegetables and grains that also went under the knife and the blessing that Allah has given you through them. They were tiny seeds that were planted and watered over time which then developed, blossomed and matured into the food you now have on your plate, all by Allah's will and by His mercy.

- **Think about WHY you are eating this food.** Is it because you are feeling sad or angry or tired or even happy? Is it purely emotional, or is it to nourish yourself so that you can gain health and energy and take care of the body with which Allah has blessed you for His sake? Is it simply because, according to your set schedule, it happens to be time for lunch or a coffee break, even if you don't feel hungry and haven't yet digested what you last ate?

Along with eating mindfully, we can also increase our efforts to source, purchase and prepare food mindfully. To do this, keep **SOUL** food on your mind:

- **S**easonal
- **O**rganic
- **U**nprocessed
- **L**ocal

When we move away from eating commercially processed and produced food, we need to take some time to re-source food, finding the best natural options available and affordable to us. Get online and google options in your local area and try to connect with others who are on the same health journey. They will be able to hook you up with any resources they have discovered, and it can save a whole lot of time getting information from others. You can also work with others and buy certain items in bulk from wholesale suppliers and then split what you've bought into smaller quantities, saving a whole lot of money in the process.

Whole Food Sources

- **Farmers' markets** – Fresh, locally produced food and likely cheaper and fresher than at supermarkets, get to know your local farmers, support 'the little guy'.

- **Weekly delivery boxes** – Farmers deliver fresh veggies once a week for a set price based on whatever is ripe.

- **Supermarkets and whole food stores** – Skip the centre aisles and head for the whole food section.

- **Zero waste stores** – Shops that have gone 'old school' where you can buy produce by the scoop and take it home in paper bags or in jars that you bring yourself or buy.

- **Online** – There are a lot of online delivery options and these can be useful especially if you live in an area that doesn't have a lot of organic options.

- **Grow and raise your own** – Growing food and raising chickens is not nearly as hard as you might imagine. You can start with a small potted garden to try it out and build up from there. If you go online, you'll find incredible examples of home growing and even more amazing examples of urban farming that is bringing fresh produce to inner city populations that would never have been able to afford it.

In Small Portions

Modern food tastes fantastic and, as we've seen, trying to eat smaller portions can be extremely challenging, so here are some practical tips to help you eat less. PICK JUST ONE to begin with, and remember this is a step process. As with anything, it takes time to make changes, and we are living in a particularly challenging period when it comes to controlling how much we eat. The struggle is real!

10 TIPS TO HELP YOU EAT LESS ONE AT A TIME

1. **Be Aware.** When you serve food, keep the one third portion size in mind. Even if you have more than exactly 'one third', you're likely to serve yourself less if you keep the reference portion in mind.

2. **Use a Smaller Plate.** Studies have shown that when we use a smaller plate, we automatically take less without even realizing it.

3. **Eat with 3 fingers.** Eating with 3 fingers will naturally slow you down, giving your brain time catch up with your stomach.

4. **Eat slowly and chew your food thoroughly.** Eating slowly gives your brain time to catch up with your body. It also helps improve digestion.

5. **Try to eat not until you're full but until you're not hungry.** This requires paying attention to your body and eating slowly and mindfully.

6. **Eat with people.** You are more likely to feel satisfied when eating with others – particularly others who are wary of portion sizes.

7. **Think of food in its natural state.** When you eat, try to think of the food in its natural state to avoid consuming excessive quantities of anything.

8. **Share when you eat out.** When you order in a restaurant, where portion sizes tend to be excessive, order one meal between two people. You'll eat less and save money.

9. **Ordering alone? Split your meal before you start eating.** Take the other half home or give it to a needy person. But don't eat all the best bits, leaving only unappealing leftovers.

10. **Portion Control for Kids.** Know what a child's portion is and don't overfeed kids. Unnecessarily large portions set them up for a lifetime of overeating. Intentionally overfeeding children, as is common in many cultures is not an appropriate way to express wealth, status and know-how; it tends to express the opposite.

WITHOUT EXCESSIVE FREQUENCY

Mindfulness at mealtime, in the context of portion control, helps us in so many ways, including helping us to accurately assess when we are ready to eat next. We may be accustomed to three meals a day plus snacks, but our body is not necessarily needy of food every time our lifestyle dictates that it's mealtime. There is a difference between real hunger and false hunger. Real hunger craves any food that will fulfill a genuine deficit in nutrients or energy. False hunger craves only specific types of food even when we are not actually hungry; our 'hunger' is only satisfied by a certain food, perhaps one with an emotional link. To tell if you are actually hungry or are feeling something different, Michael Pollan suggests taking the Apple Test: "If you're not hungry enough to eat an apple, you're not hungry."[198] When you're genuinely hungry, eat; otherwise, hold off, even if it means shifting your habits related to meal times.

Another way to reduce excessive frequency and gradually change our taste for excess in general is to follow an eating schedule that includes regular fasting. The sunnah includes examples of both weekly and monthly fasting schedules, although the Prophet ﷺ advised against daily fasting. In fasting, we seek Allah's pleasure, which is associated with reward in the hereafter, but it also brings immediate rewards, alhamdulillah. We enjoy physical benefits of fasting as well as spiritual benefits. Fasting has many health benefits and also acts as an exercise to help control our nafs. When we fast, we abstain from food, drink, and activities that are otherwise halal during daylight hours. This serves as a form of training for us, and just as fasting decreases our physical desires, it also reduces our appetite for food as well as having numerous other physiological benefits. By following this blessed sunnah, in shaa Allah, we can reap the benefits in both this life and the hereafter.

Along with reducing how often we eat overall, we can also stand to reduce how often we eat certain foods. I love chocolate, but, unlike previously, I don't eat it every day or even every week. I also, like the Prophet ﷺ, enjoy eating meat, but, to better follow his example, I have reduced the frequency with which I eat it, since he ﷺ ate meat only on occasion.

Today, eating less meat is more important than ever before. The commercial meat industry has exploded to supply a soaring demand.

Organic options are becoming available again but at a price. Eating less overall can provide savings that can be put toward higher quality meat. It is better to eat less that is good than more that comes with the risk of potentially harmful chemicals, hormone disruptors and the effects of consuming GM corn (fed to commercial livestock), which remain unknown. Eating less and better meat also means that you are not supporting the commercial meat industry's unethical production processes.

TIPS FOR AVOIDING EATING WITH EXCESSIVE FREQUENCY:

1. **Take the Apple Test** to see if you're *actually* hungry.

2. **Resist the urge to graze** on snacks all day.

3. **Increase the frequency with which you fast**. Aim to work up to fasting Mondays, Thursdays and the 3 White Days per month.

4. **Reduce meat consumption.** Start with a meat-free day each week, try out a new recipe and work your way up from there. You can also reduce the portions of meat at each meal and use meat as a flavor rather than as the focus of a meal.

DISCLAIMER

None of the nutrition advice in this book is intended to diagnose or treat any illnesses. Please consult with a healthcare provider before making any changes to your diet, especially if you are ill, nursing, have any kind of medical condition or are taking any medications.

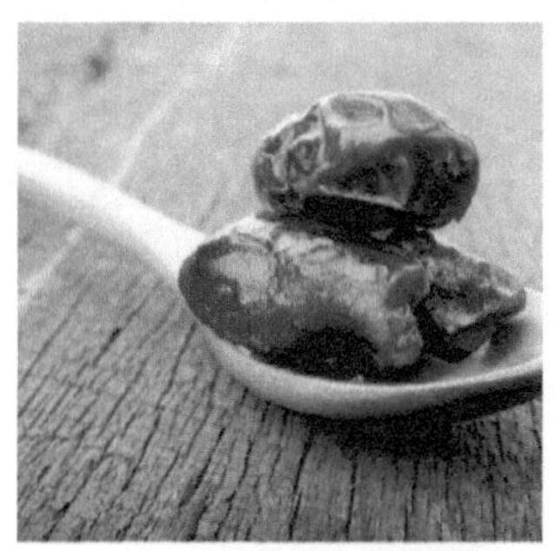

PART FIVE
MAKING CHANGES

So race to [all that is] good. Wherever you may be, Allah will bring you forth [for judgement] all together. Indeed, Allah is over all things competent. (Quran 2:148)

Chapter 28

Foundations for Change

This chapter is dedicated to Um Raqeeb and her family. This book is as much theirs as it is mine and would not have been possible without their loving support and encouragement over the years. May Allah grant her and her family the highest station in Jannah, ameen.

You may remember I asked you not to make any changes until you finished the book. One of the main reasons I asked you not to start making changes is that it is very easy to become overwhelmed. Learning *how* to make changes is as important as the decision to make them. I hope that, in shaa Allah, you have followed my recommendation and are now, as we near the end of the book, feeling highly motivated.

One thing I have come to learn over the years is that knowledge of what is 'wrong' with our food system, while a huge motivator, isn't always enough to create lasting change, and receiving so much information in one go, with so many options for change, can be overwhelming. To run out of steam in the midst of an increase in stress is a recipe for failure. So, before you start making any practical changes, let's clear a pathway and lay a solid foundation for forward movement. Please be sure to read this chapter and do the coaching exercises before you start making life shifts. If you are feeling unsure, please re-read this chapter before you begin and seek support from the growing community of those reading and improving along with you.

FIRSTLY, DON'T PANIC

As you've been reading the book, perhaps your stress has been mounting. Mine certainly did as over the course of a decade I learned how our food system has been compromised – and you've been met with all this information at once! Chances are that you're in one of three categories right now. Maybe you're motivated and mad at the food industry, and you want to throw out everything in your pantry and completely overhaul your diet. Now! And write to food producers! And tell everyone you know so they can make changes too! Or, perhaps it feels like there is just so much information, you don't feel like you can do anything about it at the moment, so switching off and ignoring the information seems like a plan. It's too much responsibility to take on. Or, maybe you are sure you want to make changes, but you also feel completely overwhelmed and even paralyzed, with no idea where to start, and you feel nervous at the thought of even trying.

When I first started uncovering this information years ago, I was a whirlwind mix of all three. Mad, motivated and wanting to change everything but also overwhelmed entirely and often paralyzed because I didn't have the guidance I needed to make positive, lasting changes. Add to that an unhealthy dose of perfectionism, and I was a recipe for disaster. Shopping became a nightmare as I started poring over the labels of food I had been buying and twisting my tongue over all the ingredients I couldn't pronounce and no longer wanted to eat. I had no idea how to navigate all the information out there or how or what to cook. I bounced around trying different things – raw diet, juicing, gluten free – each time facing a style overhaul attempting to adapt to a new way of eating. It was incredibly stressful, not only for me but for those around me as I dragged them along on my health journeys with overflowing enthusiasm, the finesse of a sledgehammer and not a lot of patience. Needless to say, I would not recommend doing it the way I did. Looking back, I wish someone had been there to help me and just say, *"Breathe. Relax. The key to health is eating natural whole food the way Allah made it in small portions. Take it step by step, be easy with yourself (and others), and here is the first step: bismillah."*

So, that is precisely what I want to say to you right now.

> *Breathe. Relax. The key to health is eating natural whole food the way Allah made it in small portions. Take it step by step, be easy with yourself (and others), and here is the first step: bismillah.*

When I was looking at the diet of the Prophet ﷺ and the example of how he ﷺ ate, comparing it to our modern diets, I could see that there is one overall principle that encompasses entirely the multiple ways in which we have gone wrong and what we need to do to get back on track.

THE KEY TO HEALTHY EATING

Eat natural whole food the way Allah made it, the way the Prophet ﷺ would have eaten it:

1. With mindfulness,
2. In small portions,
3. Without excessive frequency.

Alhamdullilah, the key to health and wellness does not lie in complexity but in absolute simplicity and getting back to basics. We do not need loads of food, variety and complicated recipes to gain good health. Rather, it lies in simple, natural whole food, and choosing to do as much as we can within our reach and our budget.

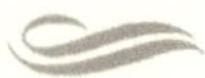

EXTENDED GUIDANCE ON MAKING POSITIVE CHANGES

AVOID A COMPLETE LIFE OVERHAUL

You may be looking at the food in your pantry and itching to overhaul. Whatever you do, do not be tempted to charge off to your pantry and fridge and throw everything out in one go unless you are <u>completely</u>

prepared in advance. Otherwise, you'll most likely have a complete meltdown when you go shopping or try to get through a week's worth of new recipes, making things so difficult for yourself in the process that even if you last a few days or even weeks, you'll eventually give up. Seriously, please don't do it. To do so would be extremism, and as such, would clash fundamentally with our deen and with the sunnah of the Prophet ﷺ. Like anything else, change doesn't happen overnight, so learn from the mistakes of others (like mine!) and do what Allah loves: *small and regular deeds consistently.*

> *The Prophet ﷺ was asked, "What deeds are loved most by Allah?" He said, "The most regular constant deeds even though they may be few." He added, "Don't take upon yourselves except the deeds which are within your ability." (Sahih Bukhari)*[199]

LEARN HOW TO EAT AN ELEPHANT

A friend once gave me bizarre but brilliant advice when I was completely overwhelmed with a massive project to the point of paralysis. She asked me, while I was in a state of mental meltdown, "How do you eat an elephant?" Unimpressed, I was thinking to my pre-Muslim, impatient self, 'I'm having a complete breakdown, and you want to talk about eating elephants!' But her answer to her thankfully rhetorical question was a life changer. She said, "The only way to eat an elephant is piece by piece."

You see, when we look at the 'whole', it can be so overwhelming and seem so impossible that we don't know where to begin, and so we stall. When we break down big tasks into tiny bite-sized portions and forget about the whole for a while, suddenly, those small tasks become manageable. As we chip away at them one at a time, those little pieces start adding up. Once we can see the whole starting to take shape, it no longer feels overwhelming.

Consider this example of a sister I know. She had mentioned to me the idea of writing a recipe book for allergy-free eating because of the journey she has been on with her children. Her doctor had been encouraging her to write the book, too, and I thought it was a great idea. I encouraged her to go ahead with it, but she said the idea was overwhelming. So, remembering my old friend's advice, I suggested a different way of looking at the project. Instead of thinking about the end result of a recipe book and all the work that goes into that, which for most people would instantly stoke up feelings of panic because they are already feeling busy and overwhelmed, I said, "Well, you are cooking these recipes anyway, so instead of focusing on the book, what about if, every time you happen to make one of the recipes, you quickly take a photo with your phone and spend just 10 minutes quickly typing up the recipe. Stash the recipe and pic in a folder and forget about it. It doesn't add much time or effort to your cooking, but, if you keep doing that, you'll have a bunch of recipes saved before you know it, with hardly any extra effort and no stress." She became incredibly excited at the new-found possibility of doing something that had just a moment before seemed impossible but was now within her reach and so easy to do.

Breaking things down into their smallest components, making them manageable, is how I aim to approach everything, and I would encourage you to do the same, not only in the process of making healthy changes to your diet, but in all aspects of your life. Being able to break things down into their smallest parts makes all the difference as we set out to achieve goals.

FIND YOUR SOLUTION IN SIMPLICITY

The goal of this book is to help us get back to a state of simplicity in our food choices, eating natural whole food the way Allah made it, the way the Prophet ﷺ would have eaten it. So much stress comes from trying to navigate all the commercially-processed food out there; it's actually far easier to start adding in natural whole food, one new recipe at a time. It does mean re-sourcing food and learning some new kitchen techniques, and this does take a bit of work in the beginning, but as with anything, the more you do it, the easier it becomes. This way, you will little by little 'crowd out the bad' and end up eating simple natural whole food most of the time and gaining health, energy, and vitality for the sake of Allah.

The aim is to simplify, working slowly, step-by-step. Even in trying to decide where to start, there are so many options, as if we are attempting to jump onto a moving wheel. Too much choice tends to produce paralysis rather than a feeling of freedom and discontent rather than satisfaction. Simplify and focus on just one thing at a time, for example, 'I want to add more vegetables to my diet, so I am going to add a salad to my lunch 4 days a week.'

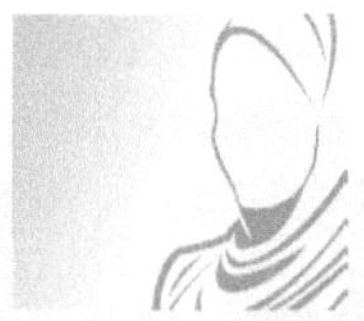

Umm Haleema

Change can be strenuous, demanding and at times unimaginable and overwhelming. These were just a few of the feelings I experienced when it was time to make some dietary and lifestyle modifications. Some of the challenges I faced included studying and researching a topic that was alien to me, abstaining from most foods at family/friend gatherings, getting others to understand what I was trying to do and why, getting over the urge to satisfy my taste buds and trying to put together meals with over half the ingredients removed. After exhausting my wits and not feeling any better I decided to see a naturopathic doctor from whom I learnt a lot of basics regarding nutrition. This new world started to feel a little more familiar and more achievable when I learnt these three basic concepts:

1. We do not need to eat as much and as often as we do, which comes from the prophetic teaching of 1/3 for food, 1/3 for water and 1/3 for air.

2. We do not need to overcomplicate foods by adding too many flavors and processes to our meal making.

3. We need to eat foods that are dense with nutrients.

Accompanying this, the doctor gave me the suggestion that one needn't feel that all the changes have to be made at once or all together. He told me to start as small as changing the salt I used to a more beneficial and nutritious one. This guidance and direction resonated with me and I began to take small steps to avoid being overwhelmed.

BUILD FOOD CONSCIOUSNESS FOR THE SAKE OF ALLAH

Much like we strive to attain taqwa (persistent mindfulness of God), we can strive to be ever-conscious of choices as we make them and of foods as we eat them. This means that instead of buying and eating without thought, we aim to become mindful of our choices, trying to make the best decisions we can. When we do choose to eat food that we know isn't 'healthy,' for we all have those days, we are better off owning that choice than switching off our mind to it – for we will be asked about the pleasures we enjoy in this life. Allah is forgiving and loves to forgive but has no interest in flimsy excuses. Likewise, we need not hold grudges against ourselves when we consciously choose to drink an occasional soda, nor should we litter our mind with a flaky defense of our actions. Allah knows of our varying needs and desires better than we know them, and He knows – He made – our ability to act rationally. Many of the connections you have with food most likely started when you were a child and are, by nature, rooted in emotion and nostalgia. If you have kids, you have the opportunity to help your children develop healthier connections with food and healthier outlets for their emotions.

We must try to be conscious of our motivations for eating and our choices. Conscious of whether we are present and grateful in the moment of each bite we take or whether our thoughts are a million bytes away? Conscious of where our food comes from and the One who has provided for us. Grateful to Allah for the plant, animal and bacterial lives that, by Allah's grace, support our survival. Conscious of the effect the food we eat is having on us physically, mentally and spiritually. Conscious of the environmental effect of the food we eat. Conscious of making the best possible choices we can. Conscious of taking small steps towards making better choices for the sake of Allah. Conscious of Allah's mercy and His reward. This act of shifting our eating from the subconscious level to the conscious can have a profound impact on our food experiences and our lives.

Sister Roshna

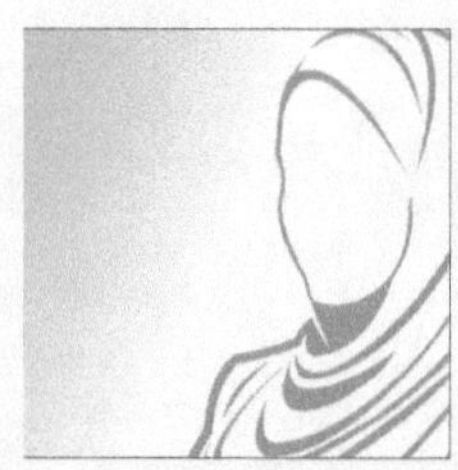

I was thinking to myself how some of us say, "Let me eat unhealthy today—I will diet tomorrow!" How can we be certain that there will be a tomorrow! So I changed my mindset, and now I remind myself every day that yesterday is gone, tomorrow is not guaranteed but I have been blessed with today to make a positive change. Allah has trusted me with His amaanah, my health and my body, and I must take good care of it exactly how Allah would want to receive it back. Positive change starts from inside. A good, healthy, natural food diet leads to healthy functioning organs and body. Just like we need food, we need spiritual nourishment to keep our heart and soul healthy which then leads to external positive changes and increased productivity.

FOCUS ON THE POSITIVE

Often, while we're doing one thing, we sabotage our efforts by thinking about all the other things we aren't doing, feeling guilty and dropping into despondency. We often tend to focus on our 'failures' or think we are 'not doing enough'. We ruminate over what we get wrong and obsess over all that we 'should' be doing or compare ourselves to others, feeling inadequate. This kind of negative thinking sabotages our efforts as it leads to despair and backward movement. Fears of poisoning your children because 'I'm not doing enough!' is not going to serve you or your children, and all those stress hormones may be even worse for your health than additives and pesticides. Focusing on the negative also leaves us feeling hopeless, it sparks negative self-talk and shaitan's whispers and we can end up paralyzed into inaction. Focus on what you ARE doing, not the things you aren't. Take it one day at a time and keep adding in little bits of good. Focus on the positive.

IT'S ABOUT PROGRESS, NOT PERFECTION

As you move forward on your health journey, know that there will always be ups and downs. That's ok. None of us is perfect. In fact, striving for perfection is not only a completely unattainable goal, it's one that creates incredible stress and serves no purpose.

In this age of social media, it's easy to feel wholly inadequate. We see 'perfect' meals, 'superwomen' doing everything 'perfectly', but we don't see the reality behind the photos. Once a 'perfect' pic is saved to our memory, it creates stress, self-judgment, feelings of low self-worth and guilt and the desire to strive for a level of perfection that simply does not exist. Even when you read a health blog, like mine, you are seeing the 'final product'. Trust me, the process of getting there was not linear. It was not smooth. It was real life, with ups and downs and challenges – and many many culinary disasters.

I cannot overemphasize that striving for perfection is of no benefit. Let's strive for excellence, yes, but we can never hope to be perfect Muslims because we are humans, not angels. We will always be prone to make mistakes, to slip, as this is the nature of mankind. If, by Allah's grace, we attain the perfection of paradise, it will be on account of Allah's perfection – not ours – and a big dose of His mercy. Just as we can strive for well-being in the hereafter without being perfect, we can strive for well-being in this life without being 100% perfect in our food and lifestyle choices.

As a qualified nutrition consultant, I would love to be able to tell you that I eat 100% organic health food 100% of the time. But I don't. If I lived on a remote organic farm, maybe I could, but the reality is I don't live in a vacuum and, most likely, neither do you. We live surrounded by food, people and choices, and we have to learn to navigate these in a way that is sustainably manageable for us. I have found it useful to reflect on and frequently recall *why* I want to make changes and *how* I want to benefit. If I choose for whatever reason to eat something unhealthy, I aim to limit my portion because I don't want to experience a loss in energy and vitality.

If you don't manage to make a particular change 100%, that's ok. Having studied nutrition, I should have no excuses, yet I have days when I don't just slip off the wagon, I tumble off and get dragged for a mile. It happens. Don't focus on mishaps because it will demotivate you, which is exactly what shaitan is working for; he wants you to give up. So, get right back up, dust yourself off, look at what you *did* manage to do, learn from your mistakes and remember, every day is a new opportunity – for progress, not perfection.

MIND YOUR LANGUAGE

Be careful of the words you use regarding food choices. We all have an inner critic who will pipe up with criticism such as, "You can't. You're fat," or "You can't, it's too hard. You've tried before and failed, so don't bother." That little voice is also sure to jump in and tell you, "You'll feel better if you have a slice of cake." Understanding this mental process, seeking refuge from it in Allah and making the conscious effort to focus on positivity and successes is key to continued motivation and positive progress. Counter mean self-talk with positive affirmations: 'I can. I am making changes already. I'm embracing health and wellness for Allah's sake. That is totally worth it."

When you talk about your food choices, mind your language. Saying "I have to give up such-and-such" implies a sacrifice (give up) that is an obligation (have to) rather than a choice by which you gain value. This creates value not for you but for the food that you are choosing not to eat. Choice of words can have a profound psychological effect. Shifting your language can shift your perception and reinforce your positive decisions. You would likely feel differently if you were to say, 'I choose not to eat this because I know that it will sap my energy. Instead, I am going to focus on eating food that nourishes me and increases my health.'

Um Raqeeb

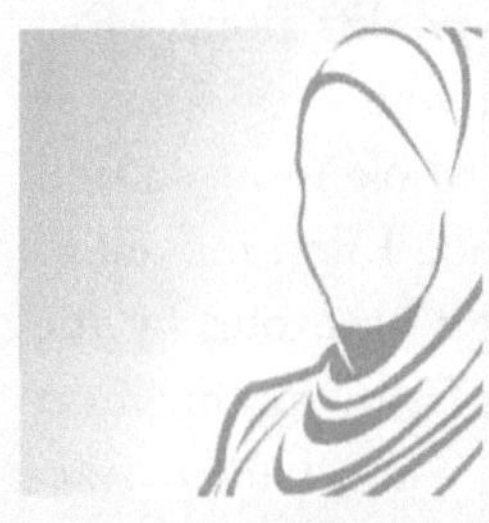

I have found the words I use with myself about food are very important. Every time I have told myself I am giving something up – I feel deprived and immediately want to eat it. I almost go into panic mode and feel as though I will never enjoy life again. So, I like to use terms like, 'I am going to allow myself a piece of dark chocolate every day.' Or 'I am going to drink herbal tea and allow myself the joy of normal tea once a day'. Changing the negative connotation of 'I am giving up' to 'I will allow myself' or 'I can't eat' to' I can have a little….' changes the whole psychology of the situation. Food should not be a punishment, rather a balanced and informed choice that allows freedom and comfort. I also make sure I savour my treat by eating it consciously and with awareness. Nothing is more irritating and unsatisfying than swallowing that piece of chocolate and not even realizing it.

Many words we use to talk about food choices suggest deviant or excessive behavior related to eating.

Having a 'cheat day' implies breaking the rules. When we make healthy living into a set of rules, it can become a constant battle of willpower. Instead, our aim is to create a positive mindset about choosing natural whole food, making it a lifestyle, not a diet, and making conscious, progress-oriented choices. When we 'treat' ourselves with foods that we know are unhealthy, we give undeserved value to unhealthy food in the form of an external reward, making internal motivation to eat healthy food less likely overall. It also suggests that whatever we are eating is something scarce, which naturally makes us want it even more. As another example, when we 'indulge' in cake, we identify cake as an indulgence, which likely sparks feelings of sinful pleasure followed by guilt, an unhealthy match. On the contrary, having a small portion of cake on occasion is ok; it makes a lifestyle of moderation sustainable. Retrain your word choices to enjoy and appreciate nourishing food.

CONNECT WITH OTHERS

We do better together, and there is no need for you to go this alone. Most likely, there are already people into healthy living in your local area, as well as farmers' markets and other sources of natural whole food, so find them and connect. It can make all the difference. When I first moved to the UAE, organic food seemed to be purely a foreign idea, but, by the end of my 10 years there, I had sourced a local organic farm, organic meat and everything else I needed. Then I moved country and had to start from zero all over again. I googled 'organic food', found a few options, got in touch and struck gold as a lovely lady got back to me with essential resources, alhamdulillah. Connecting with other whole food lovers means that I got connected with the local natural whole food supply in a matter of weeks. Trying to go it alone, it might have taken months or even years.

REAL LIFE IS MESSY AND CHANGE TAKES TIME

We all have different circumstances. Money, location, preferences, personal circumstances, current health. Take it easy on yourself and just do what you can. Rome wasn't built in a day, nor can we change our lives in a day. Remember, it's about progress, not perfection. There may be days you fall off the wagon and other times when you're totally on top of life and rocking out healthy meals. It's life. It's real. It's messy. Making lasting changes is a process and takes time. At this stage, it can seem like healthy eating is going to be a tremendous amount of work. That's what it looks like in the beginning but be patient with yourself, and others. In time, as you make small shifts, your health will improve, in shaa Allah, and at some point, you may look at the food you are eating and think, 'Wow, I could never have imagined this in the beginning. I can't believe what I used to eat. I feel SO much better!'

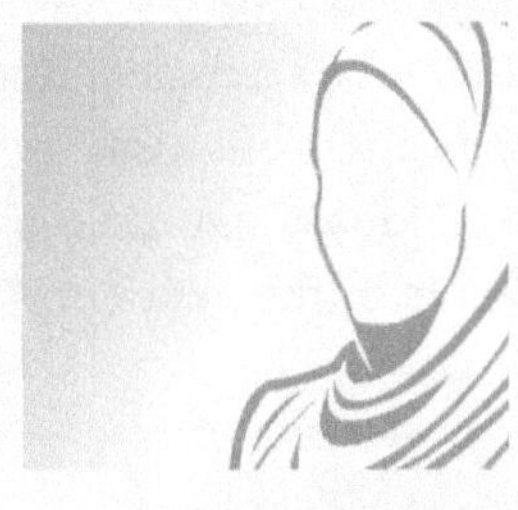

Um Zeeyad

Growing up in America in the 60's, I was bottle fed and ate the typical western diet with lots of white flour and sugar. After experiencing several health issues and having my gall bladder removed unnecessarily, I realized I had to take matters into my own hands and make some changes to the way I eat. I'm happy to say I'm not taking any medications and have lost weight and exercise almost daily. Now I feel strange when I eat poorly and skip exercise for a day. I've tried to educate myself on taking supplements, herbs, and have explored alternative treatments such as TCM and hijama. I get regular massages and would rather spend money on preventative health than lots of money on surgery and medicine down the road. I still have a long way to go and have days where I eat popcorn and ice cream for dinner, but it's only occasionally, and then I get back on track without beating myself up. Making small lifestyle changes one day at a time can make a world of difference!

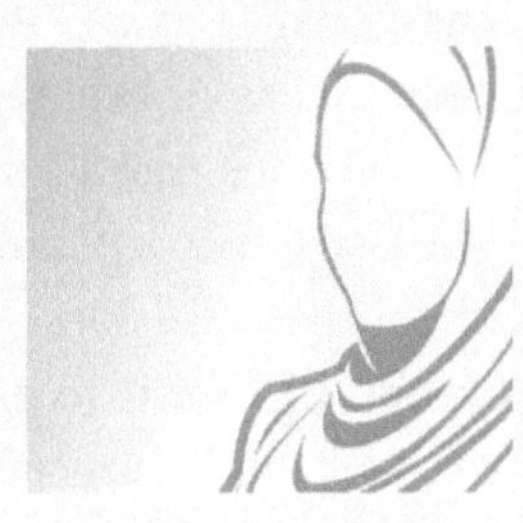

Sister Iman

Eating healthy can be challenging. The vast array of unhealthy snacks, desserts and baked goods available in the supermarket is all too tempting to resist and can take some willpower to avoid. Trying to provide healthier options for my children is how I try to deal with this problem. I make sure to stock up on fruits and veggies to snack on, and instead of buying baked goods that are full of unhealthy ingredients, we try to make healthier versions at home. Smoothies are always a hit with my children, so for me as a mother it is an easy and delicious way to make sure that my children get some good fats and vitamins. Guidance on how to provide good nutrition for our families is much needed.

SET YOURSELF UP FOR SUCCESS BY ACKNOWLEDGING YOUR LIMITS

If you are going to buy ready-made food, it's important for you to know what your limits and weaknesses are. Nobody would tell a smoker trying to stop smoking to keep several packs in the house as a test of willpower. Distractions from our goals come at us from all directions; alhamdulillah we find guidance for dealing with them in the example of the Prophet ﷺ:

> A'isha, the wife of the Prophet ﷺ, may Allah bless him and grant him peace, said, "Abu Jahm ibn Hudhayfa gave the Messenger of Allah ﷺ a fine striped garment from Syria and he did the prayer in it. When he had finished, he said, 'Give this garment back to Abu Jahm. I looked at its stripes in the prayer, and they almost distracted me.'" (Muwatta Malik)[200]

He ﷺ did not try to fight the distraction so he could continue to wear the garment, nor did he re-gift it, passing the distraction onto someone else. He gave it back. This is the epitome of wisdom.

Be honest with yourself and choose not to make things unnecessarily difficult. If we know ourselves, and know our weaknesses, we can set ourselves up for the best chance for success. I may be a nutrition consultant, but I am a nutrition consultant with a love and weakness for chocolate. It's not a weakness for sugar in general but specifically chocolate. My (pre-Islam) boss calls me Chocolate Girl to this day because of the sheer quantity of chocolate I ate while working as his event manager. It was my go-to for energy. I don't have constant chocolate cravings anymore, but I *know*, if I buy a slab of chocolate, there is little or no chance that I will eat a single square and put the rest in the fridge. There are many people who can do that, ma shaa Allah. I am not one of them. Because I know where my weakness lies, I don't keep chocolate at home. If I want to eat chocolate, I purposely go out and buy it. If I do buy chocolate, I know not to buy a large slab – just a small portion to eaten immediately. Knowing your strengths and weaknesses regarding food is an important factor in setting yourself up for success, especially in the early stages as you are starting to make changes.

Do Not Lose Sight of Shaitan's Deception and Corporate Goals

The shaitan does not want you to feel fantastic and be at the top of your game, full of health and energy and able to worship Allah to the best of your ability. If he can lead you astray and encourage you to sap your own energy through your own food choices, he will. Shaitan is not interested in your good health, and neither are most corporations selling you food; their responsibility is to make money for their shareholders, from whom they are under considerable pressure, and increased profits can only come from producing cheaper food and getting you to buy more of it more often.

Know that You Are in a Very Powerful Position

Now that you know what is going on with our food system, how the food industry works and how it is affecting you and your loved ones, remember: you are in the incredibly powerful position of being able to make choices. You have an opportunity to make positive changes every single day and, in doing so, to gain health, energy and vitality. Every change counts, no matter how small, and small changes done over time add up. If enough people make small changes over time, those small changes have the power to reform entire industries. We are nearly 1.8 billion Muslims in the world. What buying power we have as a group! A lot of it. Every time we shop, we can bring about change simply by choosing what we spend our money on. These are changes that can benefit not only our health but shape the health of our future ummah – changes for the sake of Allah that start with one simple step, followed by another and another and another.

Be the Change Your Want to Encourage

When you make health changes, you will naturally start feeling better and looking better; it will change every part of your life – physical, mental, emotional and spiritual – and people will notice and want some of what you have. Keep your success on track by being positive rather than picky, reassuring rather than showy. Lead and encourage by example, with kindness rooted in truth, remembering that you were led and encouraged by the beautiful example of the Prophet ﷺ.

Sister Roshna

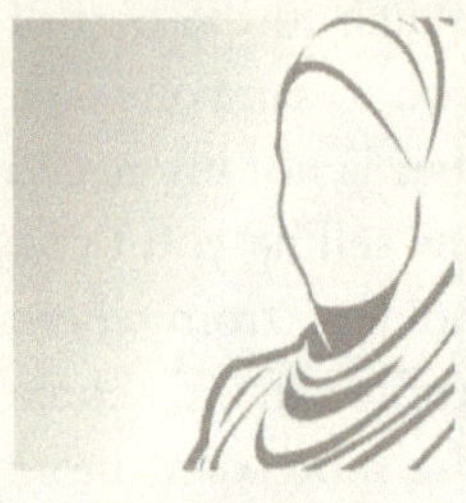

The Then and Now workshop was just simply awesome. I watched it with my family and shared with my friend. The best part is how much my children have taken in from just a short workshop. Next day we went to pick up our weekly grocery and get this - my children were very smart about what they were putting in the shopping trolley and asking themselves, "Do we need this or can we live without it?". The trolleys were full of fresh natural food and I was one proud mum with a big smile coming deep from my heart. Not once did my children ask to buy anything sugary or non-beneficial to our body, my little 7-year old was reminding me that "mummy remember cereal has hidden sugars that's bad for us" she has been eating plain yogurt with banana for sweetness.

GET OTHERS ON BOARD - GENTLY

Like inviting others to Islam, inviting and encouraging others to make healthier food choices requires wisdom, gentle speech, and patience. Lots and lots of patience. A sledgehammer approach that is unbending and critical or whipping out your soapbox at every opportunity just doesn't work, no matter how good your intentions are. In fact, there is a good chance it will have completely the opposite effect, and it can even end up causing unnecessary fitna between you and your spouse or other family members, which is not a route to any type of success. Do tread gently.

> *Go, both of you, to Pharaoh. Indeed, he has transgressed. And speak to him with gentle speech that perhaps he may be reminded or fear [Allah]. (Quran 20:43-44)*

This was the directive given to Musa and Harun when sent to reason with the King of Egypt, one of the worst tyrants in history; how much more so must it apply to us when we aim to reason with spouses, family and friends? The advice from our Prophet ﷺ is no different:

Make things easy and do not make them difficult, cheer the people up by conveying glad tidings to them and do not repulse (them). (Bukhari and Muslim)[201]

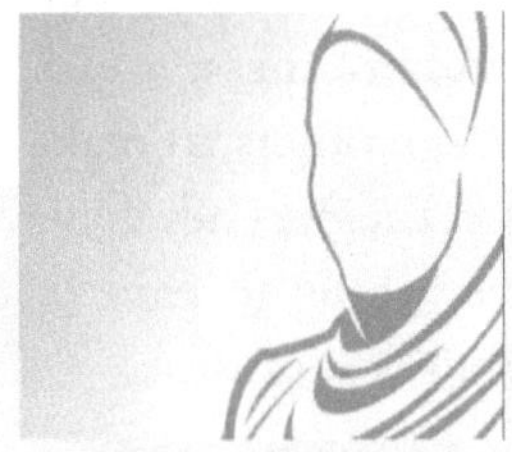

Um Raqeeb

Getting married while on my food journey proved to be a huge trial in the beginning. My husbands' idea of healthy food included pizza, burgers and kebabs. He genuinely saw it as bread with cheese and tomato, or bread with meat and genuinely couldn't understand what was wrong with it. His palate was limited, and he found a lot of new foods untasty or strange. A few weeks into marriage, I remember feeling very stressed and at a loss as to what I could cook that he would be open to and ready to eat. I knew that I had to take it slowly. I focused on figuring out what he liked and incorporating new foods alongside. I also tried hard to make sure any new dishes I made were tasty and always included salad or veggies. I tried different combinations of things to see what worked. It has been a slow process but we have been on the journey together. We both compromised on things; we didn't allow food to become a place of conflict. Food plays a role in bonding and being happy - so we focused on learning. I knew this was not an issue to force. Food is very personal and very important to each of us. Instead of me talking too much about food, I found my husband was receptive to documentaries and films. I remember one day after watching a documentary about sugar content in drinks, he announced he was no longer drinking anything but water. He has stuck to that pledge from 3 years ago and allows himself a fruit juice once in a blue moon. My husband now eats much smaller portions, he eats a diverse range of food and has almost eliminated junk food. It has taken time, but it was a positive gradual change of mindset that I know is permanent. I am extremely proud of his journey and the changes he has made for himself.

Your best bet to encourage people on board with you is to be a beacon of positivity and a walking advertisement for positive health changes. Lead by example. Invite, educate and try to bring about internal motivation within others. Speak kindly, focusing on your experience and how others stand to benefit. In the case that a serious warning is warranted, when one's health is severely at risk due to ignorance or stubbornness, it may be necessary to be firm. Be patient and try to encourage others to make positive changes because you want what is best for them. They have everything to gain just as you do, and you have everything to gain by encouraging them by way of a wise example towards a good cause.

Whoever intercedes for a good cause will have a reward therefrom, and whoever intercedes for an evil cause will have a burden therefrom. And ever is Allah, over all things, a Keeper. (Quran 4:85)

Sister Meru

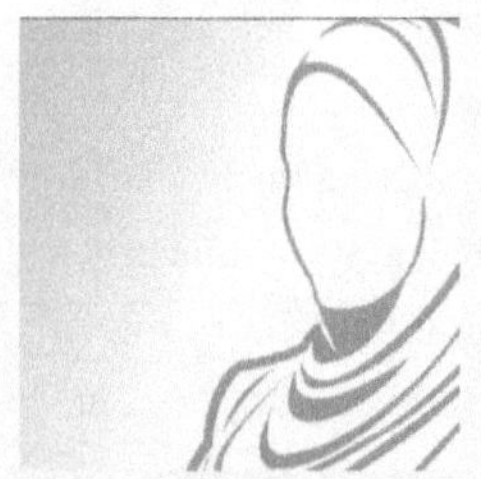

I have always been a foodie. I love to eat and I had a sweet tooth. However, I realised that the multiple health problems I'd been feeling was affected by what I ate. I had been advised many times over by concerned family members to change my diet but I just couldn't seem to do it. It's so much effort, so expensive, it won't last. Finally, I made a firm intention and put my trust in Allah to make this change. I made lots of du'a before the starting the 10-day whole food program, asking for Allah to grant me strength against my desires. I needed to cook healthier not just for myself but my family as well. He gave me more than what I asked for as my family did the program with me. We noticed changes as a family and helped motivate one another. That's right, even my husband! I was so proud of my 2 children, 7 & 9, who followed the healthy guidelines religiously. Even when they were offered chocolate they refused, and in the case of my 7-year-old, that is HUGE.

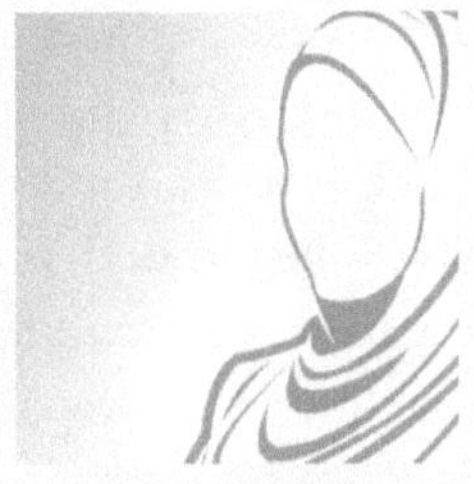

Um Hafsa

Meal prep is really fun! I made the meal plan first then from the ingredients of the meal plan I did the shopping in bulk. Then I cut up all the vegetables, separated the meat, seasoned some and packed them all in freezer bags. Now whenever I need anything I don't have to cut or chop, just take things out and put them in the pot. Saves time and makes me want to eat it. Half the time I didn't want to eat healthy because it's too much to prepare when I need something quick.

Sister Reihana

Shifting to healthy, organic and whole food items not only helping me reduce some weight, but it saved me a lot of time from shopping to cooking

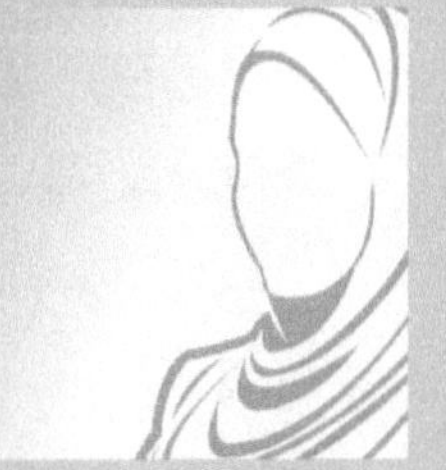

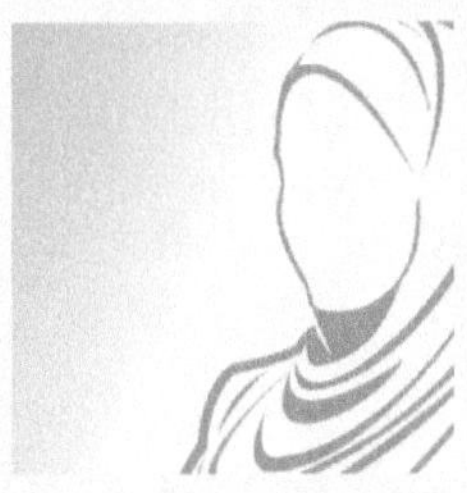

Sister Aaliya

I tried something new yesterday which I've never made before- cauliflower rice. I had chicken with stir fried cauliflower rice and vegetables- added salt, black pepper and turmeric -with a bit avocado on the side. I really enjoyed it mashaAllah!

YOUR PATH TO GREATER HEALTH

You have achieved so much by getting to this point in the book, alhamdulillah, and I hope you now have a solid foundation for understanding the deceptiveness of the food industry and an idea of some of the changes you can make, along with their incredible benefit. Step 1, developing awareness, is complete. Next, it's time to focus on intention and supplication, asking Allah to help you make positive choices and to grant you success. Once you have done that, move on to step 4, and do the coaching assessments in this chapter. These will help you learn more about yourself and your food habits, knowledge which is key to undoing unhealthy habits that you may not even realize you have and making lasting changes. Only once you have completed these, move on step 5, and begin making changes to your diet. When you start, remember to pick just one thing at a time and be easy with yourself. Continue to add in the good, crowd out the bad, substitute where you can, try out whole food recipes and re-source problematic foods. Finally, the end goal is for us to refine our choices based on whatever is available and feasible for us.

Your Path to Greater Health

Step 1: Awareness

Step 2: Intention

Step 3: Du'a

Step 4: Know Yourself

Complete the coaching questions and assessments in this chapter.

Step 5: Start Shifting to a Whole Food Diet

one small step at a time and enjoy the benefits.

> Do what you can. Don't stress about the rest. Remember, it's about progress, not perfection, and small steps add up. Don't overwhelm yourself, and don't overwhelm others!

- Crowd out the bad. Add whole foods to your diet.
- Re-source your food as needed.
- Learn how to prepare whole food – try just 1 new whole food recipe each week.
- Substitute 'less healthy' with 'more healthy', step by step.
- Learn how to work smart regarding food to save valuable time.

Step 6: Improve Your Choices Further

Continually make better decisions according to what is available and feasible for you.

Benefits of Making Changes

There are immense benefits to making positive food choices. You have everything to gain, and you, your body and your long-term future are worth it. In shaa Allah, eating for Allah and taking care of the body with which He has blessed you:

- Is a route to Allah's pleasure and a source of reward.

- Improves your quality of life.

- Increases health, energy, and vitality.

- Results in greater ability to serve others because of greater health.

- Means heightened ability to worship Allah due to improved health.

- Yields more health and energy which you can apply to doing more good deeds.

- Reduces the risk of food-related diseases.

- Demonstrates responsible character, as you won't have a hand in your own destruction through food.

- Encourages others to make better choices so that they, too, can benefit. Share the love and earn reward!

- Sets a quality example to youth for how to make better choices, therefore a means of sadaqah jariyah.

Chapter 29

Health Coaching Personal Assessment

IDENTIFY YOUR INTENTION AND PURPOSE

When we focus on eating to gain health and to take care of the body with which Allah has blessed us, eating to nourish our body so that we not only look and feel better but so we can use that new-found energy and vitality to live better, to serve others better, to worship Allah better, it changes everything. Saying no to food that we know will sap our energy and ultimately make us sick becomes easier.

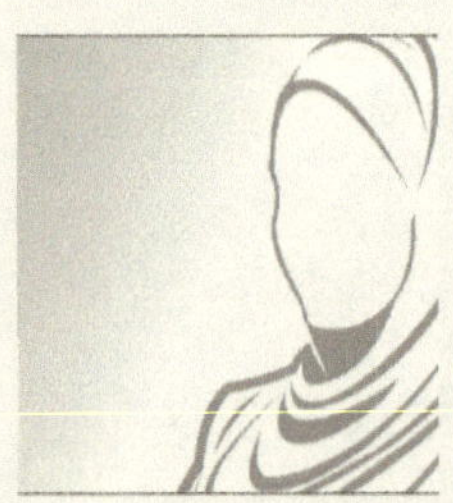

Sister Roshna

So this year I reflected back on my life, and I asked myself, who I am, why I'm here and what are my purposes because food is supposed to be nourishing us not comforting. I was focusing on temporary comfort instead of working on inward happiness which is long lasting.

Identify your purpose.

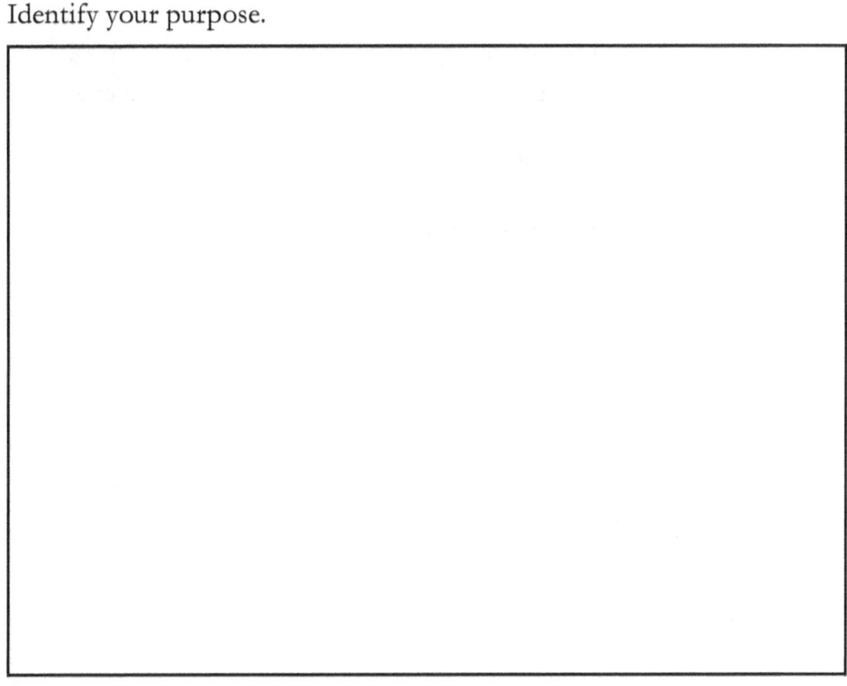

What Do you Stand to Gain?

When we have our intention clear, the mindset follows. Instead of fighting yourself, be your own ally.

Focus on why you WANT to make good choices and all the benefits you'll enjoy when you do. Don't make food choices with an 'I'm not allowed such-and-such' mindset. This gives more value to the food you're 'not allowed' and sets you up to have to battle yourself with willpower. When we mentally make something scarce (by saying 'I can't have that' or 'I'm not allowed'), that makes us right away WANT whatever we're not allowed. Watch out for similar words: must, should, shouldn't, have to, not allowed, can't. Replace them with 'I am choosing this because

I WANT greater health for the sake of Allah,' and 'I am leaving that because I choose not to eat food that will sap me of health and energy.'

Remember, it's your choice every day, and you have everything to gain.

List 5 benefits of positive change and good health.

List the benefits and drawbacks of keeping your food habits as they are now.

Ask Allah for Help

Work on your connection with Allah step by step. Allah is the One who helps us and makes everything possible.

Identify on which points you would like to ask Allah for help. Need help? Here's a du'a to start you off:

My Lord, I ask you for well-being in this life and the next. (Rabbi asalukal 'aafia fiddunya wal aakhira)

Clarify Your Vision of Health: Now and for the Future

How is your current health affecting you and your loved ones?

What has been holding you back thus far from good health?

Write a list of all the good things you are already doing for your health.

What is your health vision? What does healthy look like and feel like to you? Think about where you would like to be in 3, 6 and 12 months? Be specific.

BE HONEST ABOUT YOUR FEARS AND CONCERNS

Sometimes we don't want to try because we are afraid we will 'fail', but I don't believe there is such things as failure. Just deciding to try is courageous and is a success in itself! Every effort, no matter how small, counts and is a success to be celebrated. Even when things don't go as planned, it's ok. Instead of focusing on what we didn't do, we can learn and grow from the experience and then try again another day. You've totally got this, and you don't have to be perfect. Remember any tiny good thing that you are doing today that you were not doing yesterday or last week is PROGRESS!

I'm afraid and nervous to try because… I am concerned about…

KNOW YOURSELF: 3-DAY FOOD DIARY

The 3-day food diary involves more than simply logging down what you eat but also how you feel before and after eating, low long you take to eat, where you eat and with whom. You will very quickly be able to identify patterns between emotions, energy, behavior and food. The evidence 'on the table' may surprise you!

Download your 3-day food diary at www.healthymuslimah.com/food-diary

KNOW YOURSELF: ARE YOU MINDFUL WHEN YOU EAT?

When you say Bismillah, are you present in the moment? _________

Do you feel grateful for the food you have at the time of eating? _________

Do you sit down to eat most of the time? _________

Do you chew your food thoroughly and eat slowly? _________

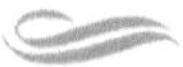

KNOW YOURSELF: EMOTIONAL EATING

A slice of cake on the occasion of Eid is not the same as a slice of cake on the occasion of sadness. The latter is a trigger for emotional eating. Using food as an emotional band-aid leads to a lifetime of overeating without helping to truly resolve the issues at the root of the problem.

Dealing with WHY we are eating, especially if our food choices are linked to our emotions, is key to making long-lasting changes. Our choices often run far deeper than simple taste preferences. Sometimes our reasons for eating are painful, complex, confusing feelings that we are trying to numb with food. Food is our medicine, but not for emotional ails! Changing what we eat often requires some deep inner work, opening and cleaning up wounds that we have bandaged with food. Journaling and similar forms of expression can also be very useful for working through emotions. If you are still struggling, it can be beneficial to see a nutrition consultant and/or other professional (life coach/counsellor) who can support you while you work through the emotional issues that are driving your overeating.

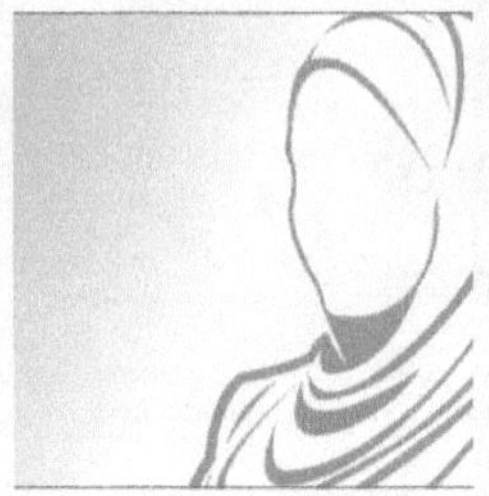

Sister Aaliya

Self-care was something I really had to reflect on, and I had to explore the many other ways I could deal with low moods and low energy levels rather than reaching for food. It is now a priority on the to-do list!

What emotions or feelings (e.g. fatigue, boredom, etc.) trigger you to want to reach for food?

Does eating take away the cause of the craving? How do you feel after you eat? How does it serve you in the long run?

What healthier, more productive outlets could you use to work through your emotions? (e.g. journaling, walking, du'a, prayer, etc.)

Sister Aaliya

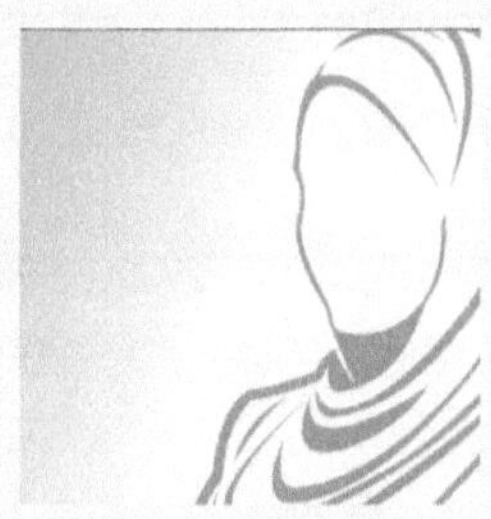

Shifting to a whole food diet while writing a 10-day journal as part of the natural eating program really made me evaluate my moods, cravings and energy levels. Sleeping when I'm tired, drinking when I'm thirsty and opting for an alternative way of self-care, rather than reaching for food to fulfil all these needs. It became more than just food and dieting and made me evaluate my lifestyle and intentions behind everything. Cooking actually felt like an act of worship, done so purely to nourish my body and energise myself.

KNOW YOURSELF: EATING FOR QUICK ENERGY AND OTHER TRIGGERS

Paying attention to our food behavior is key to making sustainable long-lasting changes. I know I make bad choices when I go for long periods without eating, don't plan ahead and get to the point of feeling starved. At that point, I am willing to eat anything in sight to boost my energy. Are you the same?

Recognizing this behavior means that you know exactly what to do and what to avoid. It means that planning ahead is key so that you don't set yourself up to make bad decisions. It also means avoiding certain situations that pose more of a challenge to us. For example, if you're trying to limit junk food, passing through the food court at the mall is probably a bad idea because the temptation may be overwhelming.

What non-emotional situations trigger you to make less healthy choices?

How will you limit these or avoid setting yourself up to make less healthy choices?

Chapter 30

Whole Food Shopping List

This list is a simple guideline for food options. It is not by any means comprehensive as there are thousands of plant and food varieties around the planet, so please add local fruit, vegetables and other natural food to this. Choose hormone-free meat and local, seasonal, and organic vegetables and fruit whenever possible. Try to eat 3-4 servings of plant-based food to balance each serving of meat.

SUNNAH FOOD STAPLES

- Black seed
- Vinegar (Raw, organic, live)
- Olive Oil (Cold-pressed, extra virgin)
- Dates
- Honey (Raw, organic)

As is the case with fruit and vegetables, try to choose meat, fish, and other food items that are in season and local to you as much as possible.

Healthful Fats
*Choose whole food fat first
Avocado
Butter, dairy ghee
Chia seeds
Coconut oil
Flax (oil, seeds)
Nuts (almonds, walnuts, pecans, pistachio, cashew, brazil nuts, hazelnuts etc.)
Seeds (pumpkin, sesame, sunflower etc.)
Nut & seed butters
Hemp (oil, seeds)
Olive (oil, fruit)
Sesame (oil, seeds, tahini)

Meat/Seafood
Organic or pastured poultry
Organic farmed or wild fish
Organic lamb, goat
Organic beef (grass fed, pastured)
Shellfish (safely sourced)

Eggs (pastured, organic)

Dairy
Cheese (Organic)
Milk (Organic or raw from a trusted source)
Yoghurt, Kefir (Organic)

Legumes/Legume Products
Black beans
Garbanzos (beans, hummus)
Lentils (green, black, red)
Pinto beans
White beans
Kidney Beans
All other beans/legumes

Fresh Fruit
Seasonal and local fruits in your area first. Imported fruit second.

Herbs and Spice Options
Basil
Cilantro
Oregano
Parsley
Rosemary
Sage
Thyme
Allspice
Cardamom
Cinnamon
Cloves
Coriander
Nutmeg
Garlic
Ginger
Mustard powder
Peppers
Turmeric

Fresh Vegetables
Seasonal and local vegetables in your area first. Imported vegetables second.

Whole Grains (and Seeds)
Amaranth
Barley
Brown rice (and other rice varieties)
Bulgur
Corn
Kamut
Millet
Oats
Sorghum
Spelt
Teff
Wheat
Quinoa and Buckwheat (technically seeds)

Chapter 31

Beginner's Guide to Navigating Labels

I am going to be honest with you. Reading labels can be a pain and can become incredibly stressful if you try to start navigating all the food you have been eating at once. How do you know what is safe, what is not – it requires understanding all the chemical labels and all the history behind them, which takes a whole lot of time and energy. Even having studied nutrition, I learned about not even half of what producers put on labels, let alone all the new deceptive techniques used for sneaking ingredients into food. I don't have the time to navigate all that, and, more importantly, I choose not to because that time would be better spent on something else. Also, I know the stress it causes; that was how I started my health journey – reading every single label. Entire books have been written on this subject, so if you really want to get into it, you can invest your time in one of those before hitting the shops.

Personally, I have taken another route. I know that 95% of commercially processed food contains ingredients that aren't healthy, so, instead of spending loads of time trying to navigate trickery, I have been buying food in its natural, identifiable form the majority of the time. That way, I know exactly what it is. Making the shift has been a step process of re-sourcing food, trying out recipes, gaining new food preparation skills and slowly transitioning my shopping list and pantry. For food that inherently requires some degree of preparation or processing that I can't do personally, like olive oil, I make the best choices based on what I know and try to limit ready-made or commercially processed food to around 10-20% of the total.

BASED ON MY RESEARCH AND MY OWN HEALTH JOURNEY, I recommend the following:

1. Buy **label-free whole food** as much as possible rather than processed food: fruit, vegetables, nuts, seeds, fish, meat, eggs, etc.

2. Learn to **make food from scratch**. Keep it simple, and it's a lot easier than you may imagine and does not need to take loads of time.

3. For food that is packaged and labelled, instead of looking at the whole and trying to eliminate, I suggest assessing which foods are most important to you and trying to **source good options** for those. Connect with people in your area who are on the same journey. Find out what they use. Once you have found options you like, stick with them and then move on to assessing another 2-3 items at a time. For example, rather than buying commercial white bread with additives, try to find a source for organic sourdough bread. For processed items you choose to continue to purchase, **see the guide below**:

BEGINNER'S GUIDE TO NAVIGATING LABELS

ORDER MATTERS

The earlier an ingredient appears in the ingredient list, the higher its content in the food. For example, if sugar is first in the list, that means that the product contains an amount of sugar that is higher in proportion to any other ingredient.

Serving Size Matters

Producers use serving size to hide excessive amounts of sugar and other ingredients knowing full well that we would naturally eat 2, 3 or even 4 times the 'official' serving size.

Splitting Ingredients - The Illusion of Less

Producers also know that consumers have become savvy and are looking for sugar in the top 3 ingredients, so, instead of using one form of sugar in a large quantity, they sneakily use multiple forms of sugar (e.g. sugar, molasses, fruit juice concentrate, dextrose, etc.) so that 'sugar' does not appear so high in the ingredient list. However, sugar by any other name is still sugar.

Fats

Consumers are increasingly sensitive about trans fats but less so about hydrogenated oils and often don't bother to check ingredients for anything other than cholesterol. Hydrogenated and partially-hydrogenated oils are just as highly processed as trans fats and are best avoided

GM

No mention of 'GM FREE' means it's very likely the food contains some sort of genetically modified product or derivative.

Low Fat Alert

Low fat often means high sugar or that other additives have been used to make it taste good.

Also keep an eye out for: 'Natural' Flavors, Colors, Preservatives, E-Numbers and Flavor-enhancers.

Chapter 32

Whole Food Action Plan

'Breathe. Relax. The key to health is eating natural whole food the way Allah made it in small portions. Take it step by step, be easy with yourself (and others) and here is the first step: bismillah.''

THE KEY TO HEALTHY EATING

Eat natural whole food the way Allah made it, the way the Prophet ﷺ would have eaten it:

1.   With mindfulness,

2.   In small portions,

3.   Without excessive frequency.

Your First SMART Goal:

With what you now know about food and the choices you have, what ONE change would you like to make first?

Set ONE smart goal for change that resonates with you right now.

Smart goals are:
- Specific
- Measurable
- Attainable
- Relevant
- Time orientated

For example:

SMART GOAL: I am going to add 2 portions of vegetables to my diet 3 times a week, and I can do that by adding a mixed salad at lunch every second day. Vegetables are a good place for me to start making changes because I don't eat many now, and it's an easy and attainable goal. I will find 3 new simple salad recipes this week and I will start adding the salads from next week, in shaa Allah.

NOT A SMART GOAL: I would like to add more vegetables in my diet. (This is not a SMART goal because it's too vague and when goals are vague, we tend to not achieve them.)

Write your first SMART Goal here:

May Allah help you on your journey to greater health and wellness for His sake. May He grant you increased health and energy and the ability to do more good with the blessings of time and energy you gain. May He also help you encourage and guide your loved ones to greater health for His sake. May every step you take, no matter how small, weigh heavily on your scale of good deeds and be a means of benefit to you in both this life and the hereafter. Ameen.

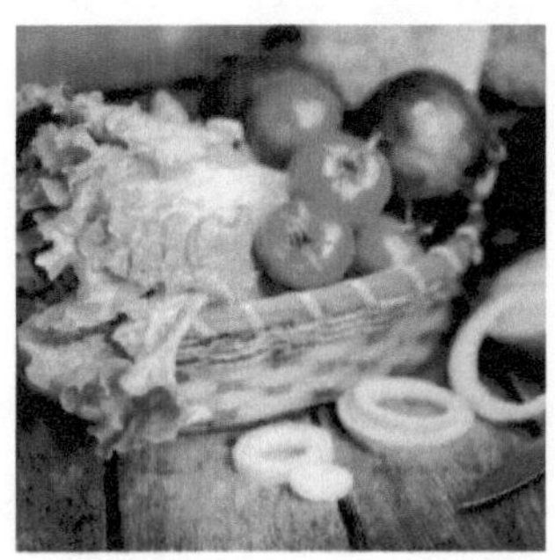

PART SIX
THE CHALLENGE

Whoever guides someone to virtue will be rewarded equivalent to him who practices that good action. (Sahih Muslim) [202]

Chapter 33

The Final Challenge

BE THE CHANGE. SHARE THE KNOWLEDGE. START A HEALTH REVOLUTION.

> *The Messenger of Allah (ﷺ) said, "He who calls others to follow the Right Guidance will have a reward equal to the reward of those who follow him, without their reward being diminished in any respect on that account." (Sahih Muslim)*[202]

If we each make a small contribution, together we could reach hundreds of thousands of people. All you need to do is tell just 4 people and encourage those 4 people to tell just 4 others. If that continues, in just 9 steps, you alone could reach over a quarter of a million people. Subhan Allah. Working together, we could transform the health and lives of thousands, in shaa Allah.

How It Works:

You tell 4 people = 4

Those 4 people tell another 4 = 16

Those 16 people tell another 4 = 64

Those 64 people tell another 4 = 256

Those 256 people tell another 4 = 1024

Those 1024 people tell another 4 = 4096

Those 4096 people tell another 4 = 16,384

Those 16384 people tell another 4 = 65,536

Those 65536 people tell another 4 = 262,144

None of us can change the world on our own, but we can change ourselves and then tell 4 people.

Be the Change.

Share the Knowledge.

Start a Health Revolution.

Visit thenandnowproject.com and find out how you can be a part of the project today!

Notes

Acknowledgement and Thanks

[1] This hadith was narrated by Abu Hurraira and can be found in Sunan Abu Dawood Book of General Behavior (Kitab Al-Adab) #4793

[2] All English interpretations of the Quran mentioned in this book come from the Saheeh International Translation of the Holy Quran.

Foreword

[3] I first heard this beautiful du'a of Abu Bakr explained in a video by Sheikh Omar Suleiman in Ramadan 2018 in the series *Prayers of the Pious by Yaqeen Institute*

1 - Duped

[4] While the details of this story have been fictionalized for the purposes of this book, the story itself is based on a factual documentary.

[5] From the documentary *Century of the Self,* 2002 documentary directed by A. Curtis.

[6] From the documentary *Century of the Self,* 2002, directed by A. Curtis

[7] This quote comes from Edward Bernays' book, *Propaganda*, 1933.

[8] This quote comes from Edward Bernays' book, *Propaganda*, 1933.

[9] From the documentary *Century of the Self*, 2002, directed by A. Curtis.

[10] This quote comes from Edward Bernays' book, *Propaganda*, 1933.

[11] From the documentary *Century of the Self*, 2002, directed by A. Curtis.

[12] This quote comes from Edward Bernays' book, *Propaganda*, 1933.

[13] This quote comes from Edward Bernays' book, *Propaganda*, 1933.

[14] The story of *Simplemente Maria* and the increase in Singer sewing machine sales has been featured in many articles including *Educating through Television* by Arvind Singhal and Everett M. Rogers available on Research Gate.

[15] *Ven Conmigo* (*Come with Me*) ran only one year, from 1975-1976. More details can be found in the article *Educating through Television* by Arvind Singhal and Everett M. Rogers featured on Research Gate.

[16] If you wish to read more on the Xerox study and Langer's work, you do so in Langer (1989).

[17] More on this fascinating phenomenon of 'fixed-pattern actions' in animals can be found in Robert Cialdini's Influence. The Psychology of Persuasion, 2014, pg 1-4.

[18] These shortcuts that can leave us so vulnerable if we are unaware of them are discussed in greater detail in Robert Cialdini's Influence. *The Psychology of Persuasion*, 2014, pg 7-9.

[19] Adapted from Robert Cialdini's *Influence. The Psychology of Persuasion,* 2014, pg 9.

[20] This quote can be found in Robert Cialdini's *Influence. The Psychology of Persuasion*, 2014, pg 9.

[21] These principles are all discussed in great details and with many fascinating illustrative examples in Robert Cialdini's *Influence. The Psychology of Persuasion, 2014.*

[22] The details of the campaign are easily found with any Google search and you can watch Edward Bernays explain the campaign in detail in an interview available on YouTube https://www.youtube.com/watch?v=WKj1W3Il85M

[23] Details of the 'A diamond is forever' campaign can be found on the DeBeers Group website itself.

[24] Found in Michael Pollan's *Cooked, a Natural History of Transformation.*

[25] "While people often choose "diet" or "light" products to lose weight, research studies suggest that artificial sweeteners may contribute to weight gain." Read the full mini-review, written by Yang Q. (2010), inspired by a discussion with Dr. Dana Small at Yale's Neuroscience 2010 conference in April that examines artificial sweeteners, their evidence concerning their effects on weight and attempts to explain those effects in light of the neurobiology of food reward.

2- A Vision of Health and Hope

[26] This groundbreaking move to ban neonicotinoid pesticides in an effort to save bee populations was well publicized in 2018, with France banning a total of 5, ahead of the EU ban of 3 of these pesticides. The details of this ban are easily found online including in *Chemical & Engineering News*, (Dupraz-Dobias 2019) and at *Organicconsumers.com*.

[27] Read more about the case of Dewayne Johnson, awarded $289 million in damages, payable by Monsanto (Bayer) in the Economist's article, *A shock court verdict against Monsanto's Roundup, August 2018.*

3 - Abundance, Excess and Discontent

[28] Read more about Schwartz's theory in his book, *The Paradox of Choice*, first published in 2004 by Harper Perennial.

[29] The report by the NRDC detailed, how America is losing up to 40 percent of its food from farm to fork to landfill, helping to spark national discussion about food wastage. Their second edition of the report was released in 2017 and can be read on the NRDC website, https://www.nrdc.org.

[30] According to a study conducted by Solid Waste Management and Public Cleansing Corporation (SWCorp) and reported in the New Strait Times as well as several other Malaysian publications in 2018, Malaysians throw away 16,688 tonnes of food on a daily basis.

4 - Just One Third (and Why It's So Hard)

[31] The English translation of this hadith can be found in Sunan Ibn Majah, Vol. 4, Book 29, Hadith 3349.

[32] These quotations can all be found in the translation of Imam Ibn Al Qayyim al Jauziyah's *Healing with the Medicine of the Prophet*.

[33] More details on the "stomach" can be found at *The Columbia Encyclopedia, 6th ed.*

[34] You can read more about the cafeteria lab rats in the study, "Overeating: The Health Risks" by Andrew Prentice M. 2001. *Obesity Research*.

[35] Read more on this research, A Behavioral and Circuit Model Based On Sugar Addiction In Rats" in the *Journal of Addiction Medicine, 2009*.

[36] Summarized from the Healthline article by Kris Gunnars, Kris. 2018. "Leptin and Leptin Resistance: Everything You Need To Know". See the article for additional detail and references.

[37] Sunan Abi Dawud, Book 28, Hadith 3836 (English Translation)

[38] Sunan Abi Dawud, Book 28, Hadith 3836 (English Translation)

6 – Processed

39 Definition of *process* from the online *English Oxford Living Dictionary*.

7 - Additives

[40] You can visit the McDonald's website to get ingredient information on all of their products including their "World Famous Fries ®: Crispy French Fries".

[41] According to the International Journal of Toxicology, Castoreum has been used extensively in perfumery and has been added to food as a flavor ingredient for at least 80 years and is regarded as Generally Recognized as Safe (GRAS).

[42] The article summarizes the history of this controversial topic and makes several very interesting interim working conclusions. The full article can be found at, *"Artificial Food Colors And Attention-Deficit/Hyperactivity Symptoms: Conclusions To Dye For"*. *Neurotherapeutics*, 2012.

[43] You can read the FDA Policy on artificially coloring oranges at https://www.fda.gov/ICECI/ComplianceManuals/CompliancePolicyGuidanceManual/ucm074540.htm

[44] Read more about this study in "Clinical Effects of Sulphite Additives" *Clinical & Experimental Allergy, 2009*

8 - Pesticides

[45] You can read the article on the Environmental Working Group Website, "Roundup For Breakfast, Part 2: In New Tests, Weed Killer Found In All Kids' Cereals Sampled", 2019.

[46] You can read a brief history and the status of DDT on the US Environmental Protection Agency (EPA) website.

[47] You can read more in Fernando P. Carvalho's review of *Pesticides, Environment, And Food Safety*, 2017.

[48] This groundbreaking move to ban neonicotinoid pesticides in an effort to save bee populations was well publicized in 2018, with France banning a total of 5, ahead of the EU ban of 3 of these pesticides. The details of this ban are easily found online including in *Chemical & Engineering News*, (Dupraz-Dobias 2019) and at *Organicconsumers.com*.

[49] "EPA Administrator Pruitt Denies Petition To Ban Widely Used Pesticide | US EPA". 2017. *US EPA*.https://www.epa.gov/newsreleases/epa-administrator-pruitt-denies-petition-ban-widely-used-pesticide-0.

[50] Read more on the study, "Brain Anomalies in Children Exposed Prenatally to A Common Organophosphate Pesticide" in the *Proceedings Of The National Academy Of Sciences*.

[51] Read more about the case of Dewayne Johnson, awarded $289 million in damages, payable by Monsanto (Bayer) in the Economist's article, *A shock court verdict against Monsanto's Roundup, August 2018.*

[52] Read more about at *Pesticides Use and Exposure, Extensive Worldwide by* Michael Alavanja, 2009.

[53] For more information, read the EPA Pesticide industry sale and usage report.

[54] The Environmental Working Group puts out its Dirty Dozen and Clean Fifteen lists every year. You can see the 2020 report at https://www.ewg.org/foodnews/dirty-dozen.php.

9- Genetically Modified Food

[55] Read more at the Non-GMO Project, https://www.nongmoproject.org/gmo-facts/what-is-gmo/.

[56] Half a century ago, India was home to more than 100,000 rice varieties with an astounding range in taste, nutrition, pest-resistance and adaptability to a range of conditions but much of this biodiversity is irretrievably lost. The article in the Guardian explains why India's farmers want to conserve indigenous heirloom rice.

[57] Read more about how scientists have used Bacillus thuringiensis (Bt), a bacterium that occurs naturally in the soil and produces proteins that kill certain insects to develop insect-protected crops through biotechnology. "Insect Resistance to Bt Crops | Monsanto". 2017. *Monsanto*.

[58] The full article and all the supporting references for studies can be found at "GM Foods Can Have Unintended Toxic and Allergenic Effects". 2019. *GMO Myths and Truths*.

[59] Information found at *organicconsumers.org*.

[60] 70-90% of harvested GE biomass is fed to food producing animals - this figure is mentioned in Alison Van Eenennaam's article "GMOs In Animal Agriculture: Time To Consider Both Costs And Benefits In Regulatory Evaluations", Journal of Animal Science And Biotechnology, with reference to Flachowsky G, Schafft H, Meyer U. Animal feeding studies for nutritional and safety assessments of feeds from genetically modified plants: a review. J Verbraucherschutz Lebensmittelsicherh (J Consum Prot Food Saf) 2012;4:179–194. doi: 10.1007/s00003-012-0777-9

[61] According to the Monsanto website, the company says, "We remain committed not to commercialize sterile seed technology in food crops. After consulting with international experts and sharing many of the concerns of small landholder farmers, Monsanto made a commitment in 1999 not to commercialize sterile seed technology in food crops. We stand firmly by this commitment. We have no plans or research that would violate this commitment in any way."

[62] Quite unbelievably, there are around 1500 varieties of mango in India of which, around 1000 have been commercialized according to http://nhb.gov.in/report_files/mango/mango.htm.

10 – Nutrient Density

[63] This quotation and more about how our soil has been depleted can be read at "Have Fruits And Vegetables Become Less Nutritious?" featured in the *Scientific American*.

11 – Sugar

[64] More can be found on the history of sugar and its effects in the journal article *Potential Role of Sugar (Fructose) in The Epidemic Of Hypertension, Obesity And The Metabolic Syndrome, Diabetes, Kidney Disease, And Cardiovascular Disease* featured in the American Journal of Clinical Nutrition in 2007.

[65] More information on this and all the references for this information can be found in the fascinating article "Origins and Evolution of The Western Diet: Health Implications for the 21St Century" featured in *The American Journal of Clinical Nutrition.*

[66] This shocking statistic can be found in the 2004 article that looks at the potential link between HFCS and obesity, "Consumption of High-Fructose Corn Syrup in Beverages May Play A Role In The Epidemic Of Obesity". *The American Journal of Clinical Nutrition*

[67] According to researchers, their research revealed that sugar and sweet reward can not only substitute for addictive drugs, like cocaine, but can even be more rewarding and attractive. You can read more about this in the 2013 article, *Sugar addiction: pushing the drug-sugar analogy to the limit.*

[68] "Contemporary research has shown that a high number of alcohol-dependent and other drug-dependent individuals have a sweet preference, specifically for foods with a high sucrose concentration. Moreover, both human and animal studies have demonstrated that in some brains the consumption of sugar-rich foods or drinks primes the release of euphoric endorphins and dopamine within the nucleus accumbens, in a manner similar to some drugs of abuse. The neurobiological pathways of drug and "sugar addiction" involve similar neural receptors, neurotransmitters, and hedonic regions in the brain. Craving, tolerance, withdrawal and sensitization have been documented in both human and animal studies. In addition, there appears to be cross sensitization between sugar addiction and narcotic dependence in some individuals." Read more on this in Jeffrey Fortuna's 2010. *"Sweet Preference, Sugar Addiction and The Familial History of Alcohol Dependence: Shared Neural Pathways And Genes". Journal Of Psychoactive Drugs*

[69] "Origins and Evolution of The Western Diet: Health Implications for the 21St Century" featured in *The American Journal of Clinical Nutrition.*

[70] This hadith can be found in Sahih Bukhari Vol. 7, Book of Drinks, Hadith 504

[71] *Then eat from all the fruits and follow the ways of your Lord laid down [for you]. There emerges from their bellies a drink, varying in colors, in which there is healing for people. Indeed in that is a sign for a people who give thought.* Translation of the Quran, 16:68

[72] There are many references to honey as a healing food in the sunnah. One such can be found in Sahih Bukhari Vol. 7, Book of Medicine, Hadith 584. A simple search through a credible ahadith source and you will discover many more.

[73] A 2017 article in Science Magazine, *Worldwide Survey of Neonicotinoids in Honey* cited that that of 198 honey samples from across the world, at least one of five tested pesticide compounds were found in 75% of all samples, 45% of samples contained two or more of these compounds, and 10% contained four or five.

[74] Read more on this and find references on the history of saccharin in Qing Yang's "Gain weight by "going diet?" Artificial sweeteners and the neurobiology of sugar cravings: Neuroscience 2010" *Yale Journal of Biology and Medicine.*

[75] Read more on this and find references on cyclamate in Qing Yang's "Gain weight by "going diet?" Artificial sweeteners and the neurobiology of sugar cravings: Neuroscience 2010" *Yale Journal of Biology and Medicine.*

[76] Read more on this and find references on aspartame in Qing Yang's "Gain weight by "going diet?" Artificial sweeteners and the neurobiology of sugar cravings: Neuroscience 2010" *Yale Journal of Biology and Medicine.*

[77] Read more about aspartame's side effects in the medically reviewed article, *"The Truth About Aspartame Side Effects"* on *Healthline,* https://www.healthline.com/health/aspartame-side-effects.

[78] Read more on this and find references on sucralose in Qing Yang's "Gain weight by "going diet?" Artificial sweeteners and the neurobiology of sugar cravings: Neuroscience 2010" *Yale Journal of Biology and Medicine.*

[79] Read more on this and find detailed references on neotame in Qing Yang's "Gain weight by "going diet?" Artificial sweeteners and the neurobiology of sugar cravings: Neuroscience 2010" *Yale Journal of Biology and Medicine.*

[80] Several large-scale prospective cohort studies found positive correlation between artificial sweetener use and weight gain in adults and similar observations have been reported in children. For details of the studies and findings, please refer to Qing Yang's "Gain weight by "going diet?" Artificial sweeteners and the neurobiology of sugar cravings: Neuroscience 2010" *Yale Journal of Biology and Medicine.*

[81] One such hadith is can be found in Sunan Ibn Majah Vol. 3, Book of Chapters on Business Transactions, Hadith 2255. A search in a reliable source of ahadith will reveal several more.

[82] In 2016, a meta-analysis was carried out to quantify dose-response relation between consumption of whole grain and specific types of grains and the risk of cardiovascular disease, total cancer, mortality from all causes. The results of the analysis provided additional evidence that whole grain intake is associated with a reduced risk of coronary heart disease, cardiovascular disease, and total cancer, and mortality from all causes, respiratory diseases, infectious diseases, diabetes, and all non-cardiovascular, non-cancer causes. These findings support dietary guidelines that recommend increased intake of whole grain to reduce the risk of chronic diseases and premature mortality. The full meta-analysis can be found at https://www.ncbi.nlm.nih.gov/pmc/articles/PMC4908315/

[83] The study concluded that in men, a diet high in whole grains is associated with a reduced risk of type 2 diabetes in men that may be mediated by cereal fiber. Efforts should be made to replace refined-grain with whole-grain foods. *Whole-Grain Intake and The Risk Of Type 2 Diabetes: A Prospective Study In Men". The American Journal Of Clinical Nutrition.*

[84] Read more in Michelle McMacken and Sapana Sha's article, A plant-based diet for the prevention and treatment of type 2 diabetes.

[85] Read more in the Harvard School of Public Health article, "Whole Grains". 2019. The Nutrition Source. https://www.hsph.harvard.edu/nutritionsource/what-should-you-eat/whole-grains/. he

[86] This hadith can be found in Sahih Bukhari Vol. 7, Book of Food, Meals, Hadith 321.

[87] Gluten's inflammatory nature as well as many other issues that we are facing with gluten grains are discussed detail in this interesting article by Ed Bauman and Jodi Friedlander. *Gluten. A Rising Concern.*. PDF. Bauman College. 2008

[88] Learn more about how to treat your grains well on the Weston A. Price website. You can watch https://www.westonaprice.org/proper-preparation-of-grains-and-legumes-video-by-sarah-pope/**15 – Oils and Fats**

[89] Narrated by Umar, this hadith can be found in Sunan Ibn Majah Vol. 4, Book of Chapters on Food, Hadith 3319.

[90] Narrated by Anas, this hadith can be found in Sahih Bukhari Vol. 7, Book of Food, Meals, Hadith 299.

[91] More details of the result of the study can be found in the review of the the evidence for effects of TFA consumption on coronary heart disease (CHD), "Health Effects Of Trans-Fatty Acids: Experimental And Observational Evidence" featured in the *European Journal of Clinical Nutrition* 2009.

92 FDA. "FDA takes step to remove artificial trans fats in processed foods: Action expected to prevent thousands of fatal heart attacks." ScienceDaily. www.sciencedaily.com/releases/2015/06/150616160256.htm (accessed January 28, 2019).

93 Read more about this in Mohammad Perwais research, "Trans Fatty Acids – A Risk Factor for Cardiovascular Disease". *Pakistan Journal Of Medical Sciences* 2014.

94 *"Season (your food) with olive oil and anoint yourselves with it, for it comes from a blessed tree."* Narrated by Umar, this hadith can be found in Sunan Ibn Majah Vol. 4, Book of Chapters on Food, Hadith 3319.

16 – Milk and Dairy

[95] These amazing nutritional benefits of milk are mentioned in the 2014. "Milk Intake and Risk of Mortality And Fractures In Women And Men: Cohort Studies" but the study also goes on to explain some of the health risks associated with milk, especially a higher consumption of milk, reinforcing again the importance of small portions and less frequency so clearly explained in our deen. Interestingly, in the study, the risk pattern was not observed with a high intake of *fermented* dairy products.

[96] Read more in "Meat, Dairy, And Cancer" *The American Journal of Clinical Nutrition.*

[97] Read more at about "Organic Milk & Dairy | Soil Association". 2019. *Soilassociation.Org*. https://www.soilassociation.org/organic-living/whatisorganic/organicmilk/.

[98] This quotation is from the online article, "Additives in Food: What Affects Your Health?" published on *WebMD*. Accessed January 30. https://www.webmd.com/diet/features/safer-food-healthier-you.

17 – Meat

[99] This is narrated in Sahih Muslim Vol. 5, Book 21, Hadith 4810.

[100] Red more on the history of meat in the fascinating article "Origins and Evolution of The Western Diet: Health Implications For The 21St Century". *The American Journal of Clinical Nutrition.*

[101] Read more on the FDA's website about Steroid Hormone Implants Used for Growth in Food-Producing Animals https://www.fda.gov/AnimalVeterinary/SafetyHealth/ ProductSafetyInformation/ucm055436.htm

[102] Read the full study on Human Health Risks Associated With Residual Pesticide Levels In Edible Tissues Of Slaughtered Cattle In Benin City, Southern Nigeria, 2015, at https://www. ncbi.nlm.nih.gov/pmc/articles/PMC5598159/

[103] As far back as 1997, an ecologist David Pimentel, professor of ecology in Cornell University's College of Agriculture and Life Sciences said that the the US could feed 800 million people with grain that livestock eat.

[104] Read the full article by Bryan Walsh "Getting Real About the High Price Of Cheap Food" at *TIME.Com.*

[105] This hadith is narrated in Sunan Abu Dawood and can be found in Riyaad-us-Saliheen Book of Etiquette of Traveling, Hadith 11.

[106] This hadith can be found in Sahih Bukhari Vol. 4, Book of Beginning of Creation, Hadith 535.

[107] Read the full meta-analysis at "Red and Processed Meat Consumption And Mortality: Dose–Response Meta-Analysis Of Prospective Cohort Studies". *Public Health Nutrition.* 2015.

[108] Read the full 2010 review and meta-analysis of evidence for relationships of red (unprocessed), processed, and total meat consumption with incident CHD, stroke, and diabetes mellitus at https://www.ncbi.nlm.nih.gov/pubmed/20479151

[109] Read more about this in "Meat, Fish, And Colorectal Cancer Risk: The European Prospective Investigation into Cancer and Nutrition" in *the Journal of The National Cancer Institute* 2005.

[110] If you want to dive into the chemistry and more detail on the chemicals produces when cooking meat at high temperatures, read the full article in, "Chemicals In Meat Cooked At High Temperatures And Cancer Risk". 2019. *National Cancer Institute.*

[111] Abu Huraira reported that Allah's Messenger ﷺ never found fault with food (served to him). If he liked anything, he ate it and if he did not like it he left it.   Sahih Muslim Vol. 5, Book of Drinks, Hadith 5121.

[112] Read more about the "Life of Broiler Chickens" in at the Compassion in World Farming website, *ciwf.org.uk.* https://www.ciwf.org.uk/media/5235306/The-life-of-Broiler-chickens. pdf.

[113] Read more about the Life Of Broiler Chickens" in at the Compassion in World Farming website, *ciwf.org.uk* and see links to the European food Safety Authority (EFSA) Report for more information.

[114] Read the original 2012 article by Cody Carlson, "The Ag Gag Laws: Hiding Factory Farm Abuses From Public Scrutiny". *The Atlantic*. There have bene further developments on the Ag Gag Laws since then with some courts ruling that such a law passed by the state of Idaho to be unconstitutional as a violation of the First Amendment.

[115] See Alicia Prygoski's 2015. "Brief Summary Of Ag-Gag Laws at https://www.animallaw.info/article/brief-summary-ag-gag-laws.

[116] See the FDA report, "Antimicrobials Sold or Distributed For Use In Food-Producing Animals". 2011. *Fda.Gov.*

[117] The CDC article, "Antibiotic Resistance from The Farm To The Table" provides interesting reading on resistance, spread, exposure to and impact of resistant bacteria. 2017. *Cdc.Gov.* http://www.cdc.gov/foodsafety/from-farm-to-table.html.

[118] See the World Health Organisation (WHO) factsheet for more information "Antimicrobial Resistance". 2018. *Who.Int.* http://www.who.int/mediacentre/factsheets/fs194/en.

[119] This hadith can be found in Al-Adab Al-Mufrad 378.

[120] Read more in "Eggs And Health Special Issue" at https://www.mdpi.com/2072-6643/8/12/784/htm

[121] Read more about eggs and cholesterol in, "Eggs And Cholesterol — How Many Eggs Can You Safely Eat?". *Healthline.* https://www.healthline.com/nutrition/how-many-eggs-should-you-eat#section2.

[122] You can give these hard-working girls a home and quality of life for the remainder of their lives by adopting then for just a few dollars through organization such as the British Hen Welfare Trust. See their FAQs for more info at https://www.bhwt.org.uk/rehome-some-hens/faqs/.

[123] Beak trimming is practiced to help reduce 'the incidence of feather pecking, aggression, and cannibalism in egg layers. Feather pecking is painful to birds and potentially induces cannibalism. Cannibalism happens in all current housing environments, cage- and free-production systems, and is one of the major causes of bird death in commercial laying hens without beak trimming. However, beak trimming has solicited a great deal of debate concerning the relative advantage and disadvantage of the practice and its impact on welfare." Read more on this study in H. Cheng's "Morphopathological Changes And Pain In Beak Trimmed Laying Hens" published in *World's Poultry Science Journal*, 2007.

[124] You can find the link to the *Model Code of Practice for the Welfare of Animals: Domestic Poultry* on the Australian RSPCA website at https://kb.rspca.org.au/what-happens-with-male-chicks-in-the-egg-industry_100.html

[125] Read the article, When and Egg Isn't Just an Egg at https://baumancollege.org/when-an-egg-isnt-just-an-egg/

[126] You can find the Muslim Homestead Group at https://www.facebook.com/groups/550286048644706/

[127] This quotation can be found in the translation of Imam Ibn Al Qayyim al Jauziyah's *Healing with the Medicine of the Prophet.*

[128] Read more about hormones and pharmaceuticals in groundwater used as a source of drinking water across the United States in the review by Randhir Deo and Rolf Halden. 2013. "Pharmaceuticals In The Built And Natural Water Environment Of The United States".

[129] "Since 2010, water utilities' testing has found pollutants in Americans' tap water, according to an EWG drinking water quality analysis of 30 million state water records." If you are in the US you can use the Environmental Working Group's Tap Water Database: What's In Your Drinking Water? as a guide to determine how safe the tap water is in your area. https://www.ewg.org/tapwater/.

[130] For more (eye opening) information on the bottled water industry, read "Bottled Water Market Share, Size, Industry Statistics | Forecast (2018-2023)" at https://www.mordorintelligence.com/industry-reports/bottled-water-market.

[131] The original video of *Peter Brabeck-Letmathe's* statement can be easily sourced on YouTube if you would like to view the original statement. The statement is further discussed on Snopes.com, "FACT CHECK: Did The CEO Of Nestlé Say Water Is Not A Human Right?"

[132] Read more about the debate on the effects on BPA in the well-researched and referenced Healthline article, "What Is BPA And Why Is It Bad For You?" *Healthline.* https://www.healthline.com/nutrition/what-is-bpa#infant-health.

[133] The FDA states that 'the safety of a food additive is not relevant to FDA's determination regarding whether a certain use of that food additive has been abandoned' and that they continue to 'review the available studies and data on BPA.' The information on BPA has been regularly updated since first being published in 2010.

[134] Read the article on PFCs at "Epidemiologic Evidence On The Health Effects Of Perfluorooctanoic Acid (PFOA)", *Environmental Health Perspectives.*

[135] This quotation by Jeff Gillman, Associate Professor of Horticulture at the University of Minnesota and author of *The Truth About Organic Gardening*, features in Dr. Mathew Hoffman's WebMD article "Additives In Food: What Affects Your Health?" https://www.webmd.com/diet/features/safer-food-healthier-you.

[136] This and other fatawa regarding permissibility of food can be found at https://islamqa.info/en/answers/118268/coffee-tea-and-sugar-can-be-harmful-are-they-haraam-like-cigarettes

[137] See the World Health Organization (WHO) diabetes fact sheet for more statistics and information.

[138] Mortality rates in Arizona differ by race and ethnic groups, and the rates appear to be worsening for most groups as seen in (Figure 12).24 in Arizona State's Diabetes Report, 2005.

[139] According to the ARIZONA DIABETES BURDEN REPORT: 2011, "Income operates in an inverse relationship with diabetes: the higher the income the lower the rate of diabetes. The Behavioral Risk Factor Surveillance System (BRFSS) data indicates that adults who made $15,000 or less had more than twice the rate (19.5%) of those who made $50,000 or more (8.3%)."

[140] See the CDC 2014 report, "Selected Health Conditions Among Native Hawaiian And Pacific Islander Adults: United States, 2014". *Cdc.Gov.* https://www.cdc.gov/nchs/products/databriefs/db277.htm.

[141] Find this quotation in Michael Pollan's *Food Rules*, New York, 2014.

24 -Gut Health

[142] Read more in Elizabeth Lipski's *Digestion Connection, 2013.*

[143] It is quite mind boggling to learn just how much of an 'ecosystem' we have in our gut. Discover more in Liz Lipski's *Digestion Connection. 2013.*

[144] Read more on the vagus nerve in Elizabeth Lipski's *Digestion Connection, 2013 pages 5, 105, 107, 243.*

[145] Read Elizabeth Lipski's 'A Voyage Through the Digestive System' for more details on the fascinating (and humbling) process that takes place when we eat. *Digestion Connection, 2013. Pages 11-25.*

[146] For full details of these, read Elizabeth Lipski's *Digestion Connection, 2013.*

[147] For more details on this, and a wealth of gut-related references to check out, read Elizabeth Lipski's *Digestion Connection, 2013.*

[148] For more on Leaky Gut, read chapter 4 of Elizabeth Lipski's *Digestion Connection, 2013.*

[149] For more on the Gut-Brain Connection, read chapter 10 of Elizabeth Lipski's *Digestion Connection, 2013.*

25 – The Creator Knows What the Creation Needs

[150] The full hadith can be found in Jami` at-Tirmidhi Vol. 5, Book of Tafsir of The Qur'an, Hadith 3149.

[151] This hadith can be found in Jami` at-Tirmidhi Vol. 4, Book of Medicine, Hadith 2041.

[152] *Then eat from all the fruits and follow the ways of your Lord laid down [for you]. There emerges from their bellies a drink, varying in colors, in which there is healing for people. Indeed in that is a sign for a people who give thought.* Translation of the Quran (16:69).

[153] Narrated Sad: Allah's Apostle said, "He who eats seven 'Ajwa dates every morning, will not be affected by poison or magic on the day he eats them."Sahih al-Bukhari Vol. 7, Book of Food, Meals, Hadith 356.

[154] Flavonoids among other plant chemicals are being studied in greater and greater depth as scientists discover the healing properties in these natural substances. Read more in "Flavonoids: A Versatile Source of Anticancer Drugs", *Pharmacognosy Reviews.*

155 Read a more detailed history in Marcus White's 2016 article in BBC News, "The Man Who Helped To Cure Scurvy".

156 Gadsby, P. and L. Steele. The Inuit Paradox. *Discover*, Oct. 2004 http://discovermagazine. com/2004/oct/inuit-paradox)

157 These quotations come from *Provisions of the Hereafter (Zaad al Maad)* by Ibn Al Qayyim.

158 I first read of the Ikarians in Dr. Jeffrey Bland's *Disease Delusion*, which then led to further investigation of the other so called 'Blue Zones'.

159 Read Dan Buettner's book *The Blue Zones* to learn more about these incredible pockets of people living (happily) to over 100 on a regular basis.

160 Liqaa'aat al-Baab al-Maftooh, 229, question no. 2 as referenced in "Coffee, Tea And Sugar Can Be Harmful; Are They Haraam Like Cigarettes? - Islam Question & Answer". 2019. *Islamqa. Info*. https://islamqa.info/en/answers/118268/coffee-tea-and-sugar-can-be-harmful-are-they-haraam-like-cigarettes

161 This hadith can be found in Sahih Bukhari Vol. 1, Book of Belief, Hadith 50.

162 It was narrated from Khalid bin Al-Walid that: A grilled mastigure (lizard) was brought to the Messenger of Allah and was placed near to him. He reached out his hand to eat it, and someone who was present said: "O Messenger of Allah, it is the meat of a mastigure." He withdrew his hand and Khalid bin Al-Walid said to him: "O Messenger of Allah, is mastigure Haram?" He said: "No, but it is not found in the land of my people, and I find it distasteful." He said: "Then Khalid bent over the mastigure and ate some of it, and the Messenger of Allah was looking at him." Sunan an Nasa'i, Vol. 5, Book 42, Hadith 4321.

26 - Our Body Has Been Entrusted to Us

163 This hadith can be found in Sahih Bukhari Vol. 7, Book of Marriage, Hadith 127.

164 This hadith can be found in Sahih al-Bukhari Vol. 8, Book of Softening the Heart, Hadith 425 and the narration including the sub narrating can also be found in well-known compilation of Nawawi's Forty Hadith.

165 *Narrated by Sahih Bukhari in al-Adab al-Mufrad (300) and by al-Tirmidhi in al-Sunan (2346)/; hasan ghareeb.*

166 This hadith can be found in Sahih Bukhari Vol. 8, Book of Softening the Heart, Hadith 421.

167 This hadith can be found in Tirmidhi Vol. 6, Book of Tafsir Of The Qur'an, Hadith 3358.

168 This hadith is classed as da'if in Tirmidhi and later classed as hasan by al-Albaani in Saheeh al-Tirmidhi, 1969. While all of the other ahadith mentioned so far are classed sahih, I thought it worth including this as the principle of personal accountability when it comes to our health is key in understanding the importance of taking care of our bodies as an amaanah.

169 Saheeh al Jaami' no. 1077 referenced in https://islamqa.info/en/answers/47398/how-should-a-person-fill-his-spare-time.

[170] The details of too much eating being one of the poisons of the heart can be found on pg 29-30 of *Purification of the Soul*, a compilation of the works of Ibn Rajab al Hanbali, Ibn Al Qayyim and Abu Hamid al-Ghazali.

[171] Tareeq al-Hijratayn, 1/460 referenced in https://islamqa.info/en/answers/4094/dealing-with-evil-within-oneself

[172] Uddat al-Saabireen, 1/46 referenced in https://islamqa.info/en/answers/4094/dealing-with-evil-within-oneself

[173] A man said: O Messenger of Allah, should I tie up [my camel] and rely on Allah, or should I leave it loose and rely on Him? He said: "Tie it up and rely [on Allah]."Narrated by at-Tirmidhi (2517); classed as hasan by al-Albaani in Saheeh Sunan at-Tirmidhi (2/610). Retrieved from https://islamqa.info/en/answers/270017/is-it-obligatory-to-entrust-all-our-affairs-to-allah

27 – How the Prophet ﷺ Ate

[174] This comes from *Provisions of the Hereafter (Zaad al Maad)* by Ibn Al Qayyim *Zaad al-Ma'aad (1/147) sources in https://islamqa.info/en/answers/102374/ahaadeeth-of-the-prophet-peace-and-blessings-of-allaah-be-upon-him-which-criticize-extravagance-with-regard-to-food*

[175] Narrated Jabir that the Prophet (ﷺ) said: "What an excellent condiment vinegar is." – this hadith can be found in Jami' at-Tirmidhi Vol. 3, Book of Food, Hadith 1839 and a search on the word 'vinegar' in a reputable online ahadith website will yield dozens more examples.

[176] This hadith can be found in Jami' at-Tirmidhi Vol. 4, Book of Medicine, Hadith 2041.

[177] It was narrated from 'Umar that the Messenger of Allah (Peace be upon him) said: 'Season (your food) with olive oil and anoint yourselves with it, for it comes from a blessed tree." Sunan Ibn Majah Vol. 4, Book of Chapters on Food, Hadith 3319.

[178] There are many references to honey as a healing food in the sunnah. One such can be found in Sahih Bukhari Vol. 7, Book of Medicine, Hadith 584. A simple search through a credible ahadith source and you will discover many more. Allah also speaks of the healing benefits of honey in the *Quran (16:69)*.

[179] Narrated Sad: Allah's Apostle said, "He who eats seven 'Ajwa dates every morning, will not be affected by poison or magic on the day he eats them."Sahih al-Bukhari Vol. 7, Book of Food, Meals, Hadith 356.

[180] This hadith is featured in Riyadh au-Saliheen (Gardens of the Righteous) as one narrated in both Sahih Bukhari and Sahih Muslim.

[181] This hadith can be found in Jami' at-Tirmidhi Vol. 4, Book of Zuhd, Hadith 2380.

[182] This hadith can be found in Sahih Muslim Vol. 5, Book of Drinks, Hadith 5112.

[183] This hadith can be found in Sahih Muslim Vol. 5, Book of Drinks, Hadith 5040.

[184] This hadith can be found in Sahih al-Bukhari Vol. 7, Book of Food, Meals, Hadith 342.

[185] This hadith can be found in Sahih Muslim Vol. 5, Book of Drinks, Hadith 5029.

[186] This hadith can be found in Sunan an Nasaa'i, Vol. 5, Book 42, Hadith 4321

[187] This hadith can be found in Sunan Abu Dawood Vol. 4, Book of Foods (Kitab Al-Atimah), Hadith 3755. Though it is classed as hasan, I thought it most relevant especially in light of our modern trend to eat alone or on the run.

[188] This hadith is from Sahih Bukhari and is mentioned in Riyaad-us-saliheen Book of Etiquette of Eating, Hadith 19.

[189] This hadith can be found in Sahih al-Bukhari Vol. 4, Book of Merits of Sunnah, Hadith 764.

[190] This hadith can be found in Sahih Muslim Vol. 5, Book of Drinks, Hadith 5049.

[191] Anas reported that when Allah's Messenger (Peace be upon him) ate food he licked his three fingers, and he said: "When any one of you drops a mouthful he should remove anything filthy from it and then eat it, and should not leave it for the Satan." He also commanded us that we should wipe the dish saying, "You do not know in what portion of your food the blessing lies."

[192] The full hadith can be found in Sahih Muslim Vol. 5, Book of Drinks, Hadith 5070.

[193] This hadith can be found in Riyaad-us-saliheen Book of Virtues, Hadith 267.

[194] This hadith can be found in Sunan Abu Dawood Vol. 3, Book of Fasting (Kitab Al-Siyam), Hadith 2443.

[195] This hadith can be found in Sahih al-Bukhari Vol. 3, Book of Fasting, Hadith 146.

[196] This hadith can be found in Sahih al-Bukhari Vol. 3, Book of Fasting, Hadith 178.

[197] This hadith can be found in   Sunan an-Nasaa'i Vol. 3, Book of Fasting, Hadith 2401.

[198] The apple test can be found in Michael Pollan's 2014. *Food Rules*. New York: Penguin Books.

28 – Foundations for Change

[199] This hadith can be found in Sahih al-Bukhari Vol. 8, Book of Softening the Heart, Hadith 472.

[200] This can be found in Muwatta Malik Book of Prayer, Hadith 72. I was not able to find any classification of the hadith.

[201] This hadith can be found in both Sahih Bukhari and Sahih Muslim and is featured in Riyaad-us-saliheen Book of Miscellany, Hadith 637.

33 – The Final Challenge

[202] This hadith can be found is Sahih Muslim and is featured in Riyaad-us-saliheen Book of Miscellany, Hadith 173.

Bibliography

Abid, Zaynah, Amanda J Cross, and Rashmi Sinha. 2014. "Meat, Dairy, and Cancer". *The American Journal of Clinical Nutrition*, 100 (suppl_1): 386S-393S. doi:10.3945/ajcn.113.071597.

Alavanja, Michael C. R. 2009. "Introduction: Pesticides Use and Exposure, Extensive Worldwide". *Reviews on Environmental Health*, 24 (4). doi:10.1515/reveh.2009.24.4.303.

Al Jauziyah, Ibn Al Qayyim. *Healing with the Medicine of the Prophet*. English Translation. Darusalaam Publishers.

Al Jauziyah, Ibn Al Qayyim. *Provisions of the Hereafter*. English Translation. Darussalaam Publishers.

Ahmed, Serge H., Karine Guillem, and Youna Vandaele. 2013. "Sugar Addiction. Pushing the Drug Sugar Addiction Analogy to the Limit". *Current Opinion in Clinical Nutrition and Metabolic Care*, 16 (4): 434-439. doi:10.1097/mco.0b013e328361c8b8.

Arnold, L. Eugene, Nicholas Lofthouse, and Elizabeth Hurt. 2012. "Artificial Food Colors And Attention-Deficit/Hyperactivity Symptoms: Conclusions To Dye For". *Neurotherapeutics*, 9 (3): 599-609. doi:10.1007/s13311-012-0133-x.

Aune, Dagfinn, NaNa Keum, Edward Giovannucci, Lars T Fadnes, Paolo Boffetta, Darren C Greenwood, Serena Tonstad, Lars J Vatten, Elio Riboli, and Teresa Norat. 2016. "Whole Grain Consumption and Risk of Cardiovascular Disease, Cancer, and All Cause and Cause Specific Mortality: Systematic Review and Dose-Response Meta-Analysis of Prospective Studies". *BMJ*, i2716. doi:10.1136/bmj.i2716.

Bauman, Ed, and Jodi Friedlander. 2008. *Gluten: A Rising Concern*. Ebook. Bauman College.

Bernays, Edward. "Bacon and Eggs for Breakfast". Interview with Edward Bernays. https://www.youtube.com/watch?v=WKj1W3lI85M

Bernays, Edward L. 2005. *Propaganda*. (Reprint) New York: Liveright Ig Publishing.

Bland, Jeffrey. 2014. *The Disease Delusion*. Harper Collins.

Bray, George A, Samara Joy Nielsen, and Barry M Popkin. 2004. "Consumption of High-Fructose Corn Syrup In Beverages May Play A Role In The Epidemic Of Obesity". *The American Journal of Clinical Nutrition*, 79 (4): 537-543. doi:10.1093/ajcn/79.4.537.

Burdock, G. A. 2007. "Safety Assessment Of Castoreum Extract As A Food Ingredient". *International Journal of Toxicology*, 26 (1): 51-55. doi:10.1080/10915810601120145.

Carlson, Cody. 2012. "The Ag Gag Laws: Hiding Factory Farm Abuses From Public Scrutiny". *The Atlantic*. https://www.theatlantic.com/health/archive/2012/03/the-ag-gag-laws-hiding-factory-farm-abuses-from-public-scrutiny/254674/.

Carvalho, Fernando P. 2017. "Pesticides, Environment, and Food Safety". *Food and Energy Security*, 6 (2): 48-60. doi:10.1002/fes3.108.

Century of the Self. 2002. [film] Directed by A. Curtis.

Cheng, H. 2007. "Morphopathological Changes And Pain In Beak Trimmed Laying Hens". *World's Poultry Science Journal*, 62 (01): 41-52. doi:10.1079/wps200583.

Choudhury, Chitrangada. 2017. "Why India's Farmers Want to Conserve Indigenous Heirloom Rice". *The Guardian*. https://www.theguardian.com/environment/2017/sep/24/why-indias-farmers-want-to-conserve-indigenous-heirloom-rice.

Cialdini, Robert B. 2014. *Influence*. Harlow: Pearson Education.

Cordain, Loren, S Boyd Eaton, Anthony Sebastian, Neil Mann, Staffan Lindeberg, Bruce A Watkins, James H O'Keefe, and Janette Brand-Miller. 2005. "Origins and Evolution of the Western Diet: Health Implications for the 21st Century". *The American Journal of Clinical Nutrition*, 81 (2): 341-354. doi:10.1093/ajcn.81.2.341.

Deo, Randhir, and Rolf Halden. 2013. "Pharmaceuticals in the Built And Natural Water Environment of the United States". *Water*, 5 (3): 1346-1365. doi:10.3390/w5031346.

Dupraz-Dobias, Paula. 2019. "France Bans All Uses Of Neonicotinoid Pesticides, Outpacing European Union Measure". *Chemical & Engineering News*. https://cen.acs.org/environment/pesticides/France-bans-uses-neonicotinoid-pesticides/96/i36

Farid, Ahmed, Ed. 1991. *Purification of the Soul*. Compilation of the works of Ibn Rajab al Hanbali, Ibn Al Qayyim and Abu Hamid al-Ghazali. London: Al Firdaus Ltd.

Fernandez, Maria. 2016. "Eggs and Health Special Issue". *Nutrients*, 8 (12): 784. doi:10.3390/nu8120784.

Fortuna, Jeffrey L. 2010. "Sweet Preference, Sugar Addiction and the Familial History of Alcohol Dependence: Shared Neural Pathways and Genes". *Journal of Psychoactive Drugs*, 42 (2): 147-151. doi:10.1080/02791072.2010.10400687.

Fung, Teresa T, Frank B Hu, Mark A Pereira, Simin Liu, Meir J Stampfer, Graham A Colditz, and Walter C Willett. 2002. "Whole-Grain Intake and the Risk of Type 2 Diabetes: A Prospective Study in Men". *The American Journal of Clinical Nutrition*, 76 (3): 535-540. doi:10.1093/ajcn/76.3.535.

Galinsky, Adena M., Carla E. Zelaya, Patricia M. Barnes, and Catherine Simile. 2014. "Selected Health Conditions Among Native Hawaiian and Pacific Islander Adults". https://www.cdc.gov/nchs/products/databriefs/db277.htm.

Gunders, Dana. 2017. "Wasted: How America Is Losing Up To 40 Percent Of Its Food From Farm To Fork To Landfill". NRDC. https://www.nrdc.org/resources/wasted-how-america-losing-40-percent-its-food-farm-fork-landfill.

Gunnars, Kris. 2018. "Eggs And Cholesterol — How Many Eggs Can You Safely Eat?". *Healthline.* https://www.healthline.com/nutrition/how-many-eggs-should-you-eat#section2.

Gunnars, Kris. 2018. "Leptin And Leptin Resistance: Everything You Need To Know". *Healthline.* https://www.healthline.com/nutrition/leptin-101#section3.

Healthline editorial team. "The Truth About Aspartame Side Effects". 2019. *Healthline.* https://www.healthline.com/health/aspartame-side-effects.

Hoebel, Bartley G., Nicole M. Avena, Miriam E. Bocarsly, and Pedro Rada. 2009. "A Behavioral and Circuit Model Based on Sugar Addiction in Rats". *Journal of Addiction Medicine*, 3 (1). doi:10.1097/adm.0b013e31819aa621.

Hoffman, Mathew. 2019. "Additives In Food: What Affects Your Health?". WebMD. https://www.webmd.com/diet/features/safer-food-healthier-you.

Iqbal, Mohammad Perwaiz. 2014. "Trans Fatty Acids – A Risk Factor For Cardiovascular Disease". *Pakistan Journal of Medical Sciences*, 30 (1). doi:10.12669/pjms.301.4525.

Johnson, Richard, Mark Segal, Yuri Sautin, Takahiko Nakagawa, Daniel Feig, Duk-Hee Kang, Michael Gersch, Steven Benner, and Laura Sánchez-Lozada 2007. "Potential Role of Sugar (Fructose) in the Epidemic of Hypertension, Obesity and the Metabolic Syndrome, Diabetes, Kidney Disease, and Cardiovascular Disease". *The American Journal of Clinical Nutrition*, 86 (4).

Langer, Ellen J. 1989. *Mindfulness.* Reading, Mass.: Addison-Wesley Pub. Co.

Lipski, Elizabeth. 2013. *Digestion Connection.* Exclusive Expanded Edition. Rodale.

McLinn, Jason. 2018. "A Shock Court Verdict Against Monsanto's Roundup". *The Economist.* https://www.economist.com/business/2018/08/18/a-shock-court-verdict-against-monsantos-roundup.

McMacken, Michelle and Sapana Shah. 2017. "A plant-based diet for the prevention and treatment of type 2 diabetes". *Journal of Geriatric Cardiology*, 14 (5). 342-354.

Micha, Renata, Sarah K. Wallace, and Dariush Mozaffarian. 2010. "Red and Processed Meat Consumption and Risk of Incident Coronary Heart Disease, Stroke, and Diabetes Mellitus". *Circulation*, 121 (21): 2271-2283. doi:10.1161/circulationaha.109.924977.

Michaelsson, K., A. Wolk, S. Langenskiold, S. Basu, E. Warensjo Lemming, H. Melhus, and L. Byberg. 2014. "Milk Intake and Risk of Mortality and Fractures in Women and Men: Cohort Studies". *BMJ*, 349 (Oct. 27): g6015-g6015. doi:10.1136/bmj.g6015.

Mitchell, E. A. D., B. Mulhauser, M. Mulot, A. Mutabazi, G. Glauser, and A. Aebi. 2017. "A Worldwide Survey of Neonicotinoids in Honey". *Science* 358 (6359): 109-111. doi:10.1126/science.aan3684.

Mozaffarian, D, A Aro, and W C Willett. 2009. "Health Effects of Trans-Fatty Acids: Experimental and Observational Evidence". *European Journal of Clinical Nutrition*, 63 (S2): S5-S21. doi:10.1038/sj.ejcn.1602973.

Norat, Teresa, Sheila Bingham, Pietro Ferrari, Nadia Slimani, Mazda Jenab, Mathieu Mazuir, and Kim Overvad et al. 2005. "Meat, Fish, and Colorectal Cancer Risk: The European Prospective Investigation into Cancer and Nutrition". *Journal Of The National Cancer Institute*, 97 (12): 906-916. doi:10.1093/jnci/dji164.

Petre, Alina. 2018. "What Is BPA And Why Is It Bad For You?". *Healthline.* https://www.healthline.com/nutrition/what-is-bpa#infant-health.

Pollan, Michael. 2013. *A Natural History of Transformation*. London: Allen Lane.

Pollan, Michael. 2014. *Food Rules*. New York: Penguin Books.

Pope, Sarah. 2011. "Proper Preparation Of Grains And Legumes". [Video] The Weston A. Price Foundation. https://www.westonaprice.org/proper-preparation-of-grains-and-legumes-video-by-sarah-pope/.

Prentice, Andrew M. 2001. "Overeating: The Health Risks". *Obesity Research*, 9 (S11): 234S-238S. doi:10.1038/oby.2001.124.

Prygoski, Alicia. 2015. "Brief Summary Of Ag-Gag Laws". Animal Legal & Historical Center. https://www.animallaw.info/article/brief-summary-ag-gag-laws.

Rauh, V. A., F. P. Perera, M. K. Horton, R. M. Whyatt, R. Bansal, X. Hao, J. Liu, D. B. Barr, T. A. Slotkin, and B. S. Peterson. 2012. "Brain Anomalies In Children Exposed Prenatally To A Common Organophosphate Pesticide". *Proceedings of the National Academy of Sciences*, 109 (20): 7871-7876. doi:10.1073/pnas.1203396109.

Samuel, Henry. 2019. "France Becomes First Country In Europe To Ban All Five Pesticides Killing Bees". https://www.organicconsumers.org/news/france-becomes-first-country-europe-ban-all-five-pesticides-killing-bees#close.

Scheer, Roddy and Doug Moss. 2019. "Dirt Poor: Have Fruits And Vegetables Become Less Nutritious?" *Scientific American*. https://www.scientificamerican.com/article/soil-depletion-and-nutrition-loss/.

Schwartz, Barry. 2004. *The Paradox of Choice*. Harper Perennial.

Sharma, Neelu, MahabeerP Dobhal, YogeshC Joshi, and MaheepK Chahar. 2011. "Flavonoids: A Versatile Source of Anticancer Drugs". *Pharmacognosy Reviews*, 5 (9): 1. doi:10.4103/0973-7847.79093.

Singhal, Arvind & M Rogers, Everett. (1989). Educating through television. *Populi*. 16.

Steenland, Kyle, Tony Fletcher, and David A. Savitz. 2010. "Epidemiologic Evidence On The Health Effects Of Perfluorooctanoic Acid (PFOA)". *Environmental Health Perspectives*, 118 (8): 1100-1108. doi:10.1289/ehp.0901827.

Suleiman, Omar. "Make me better than what they think." Prayers of the Pious Ramadan Series. Video series, episode 19. https://yaqeeninstitute.org/en/omar-suleiman/episode-19-make-me-better-than-what-they-think-prayers-of-the-pious-ramadan-series/

Tongo, Isioma, and Lawrence Ezemonye. 2015. "Human Health Risks Associated With Residual Pesticide Levels In Edible Tissues Of Slaughtered Cattle In Benin City, Southern Nigeria". *Toxicology Reports*, 2: 1117-1135. doi:10.1016/j.toxrep.2015.07.008.

Vally, H., N. L. A. Misso, and V. Madan. 2009. "Clinical Effects Of Sulphite Additives". *Clinical & Experimental Allergy*, 39 (11): 1643-1651. doi:10.1111/j.1365-2222.2009.03362.x.

Van Eenennaam, Alison L. 2013. "Gmos In Animal Agriculture: Time To Consider Both Costs And Benefits In Regulatory Evaluations". *Journal of Animal Science and Biotechnology*, 4 (1). doi:10.1186/2049-1891-4-37.

Walsh, Bryan. 2009. "Getting Real About The High Price Of Cheap Food". *TIME.Com*. http://content.time.com/time/subscriber/article/0,33009,1917726-1,00.html.

Wang, Xia, Xinying Lin, Ying Y Ouyang, Jun Liu, Gang Zhao, An Pan, and Frank B Hu. 2015. "Red And Processed Meat Consumption And Mortality: Dose–Response Meta-Analysis Of Prospective Cohort Studies". *Public Health Nutrition*, 19 (05): 893-905. doi:10.1017/s1368980015002062.

White, Marcus. 2016. "The Man Who Helped To Cure Scurvy". *BBC News*. https://www.bbc.com/news/uk-england-37320399.

Yang, Q. 2010. "Gain weight by 'going diet'? Artificial sweeteners and the neurobiology of sugar cravings". *The Yale Journal of Biology and Medicine*, 83(2), 101-8.

Index

Abundance
  Allah's creation, 80, 83
  and excess 39 - 45
  and variety 41
  Fatty fish 154
  Food, 156, 173
  Overabundance, Paradox of Choice 43
  Perpetual abundance 52
Addicted/Addiction 56, 91
Additives 64
  Aspartame 96
  Castoreum 66
  Colors 67-68
  Cyclamate 96
  Flavors and Flavor Enhancers 66-67
  High Fructose Corn Syrup 30, 60, 67, 89
  MacDonald's fries 66
  MSG, monosodium glutamate 67
  Navigating 69
  Neotame 96
  Preservatives 68-69
  Saccharin 96
  Sucralose 96
  Sweeteners (artificial) 67, 95-97
  Sulfites 68
ADHD 81
Allah's Mercy 196

American Heart Association 123
Antibiotics
  Antibiotic free food 174
  Chicken 119-120, 127
  Fish 129
  Gut health and antibiotics 148
  Milk and dairy 109-110
  Meat 113
Anxiety 56, 140, 150
Apple Test 188
Artificial Sweeteners (see additives)
Aspartame (see additives)
Asthma 69
Bacon and eggs 25
Bernays, Edward 18 - 20, 22, 25
Black seed 152, 176,
Blue Zones 155
BPA
  BPA-free packaging 34
  Diabetes 135
  Health effects 135-136
  Water purity 132
Brabeck-Letmathe, Peter 132-133
Breakfast 89
Bt corn 81
Buettner, Dan (Blue Zones) 155
Butter 105, 107, 153

Cancer 17, 30
  GM 81
    Hawaiians 144
    Hormones in milk 109
    Lower risk (wholegrains) 98
    Meat 115-116
    Monsanto Court Case 33, 74
    Pesticides 72
    Sweeteners 96
Cardiovascular disease
  Lower risk (wholegrains) 98
  Margarine/Trans fat link 105,153
  Meat 115
  Overeating 48
  Poor food choices 30
  Standard Modern Diet (SMD) 17
Cereal 41
  Common 'healthy' breakfast 89
  Containing pesticides 71
  Hidden sugar 89
Challenge, Final 230
Chia, Kale, and Blueberries 158
Chicken 118 - 122
  Action points 121
  Antibiotics and feed (see antibiotics)
  Broiler 118-119
  Conscientious consumers 29-30, 31
  Culling of male chicks 125
  De-beaking 124-125
  Disconnected from food supply 42, 53
  Eggs 123 - 127
  Ethics 120 - 121
  Know your chickens 120
Chlorpyrifos (see pesticides)
Cholesterol 100
  Eggs 123-124
Cialdini, Robert 21-25
Cigarette sales 19
Cocaine (sugar addiction) 91
Compliant Consumers 26, 32
Consumer behavior 21-30
Cyclamate (see additives)
Dates 177
  Ajwa 153
  Excess and harm 141, 159-160
DDT (see pesticides)
De-beaking (see chickens)

DeBeers Group 26
Depression
  Total load 140
  Gut health 147, 149-150
Dewayne Lee Johnson (court case) 74
Diabetes
  BPA (see BPA)
  Hawaiians 144
  Muslim countries 144
  Rates increasing 143
Diamonds 26
Digestion 90, 85
  The Process 146-148
  Issues/problems 146, 148
  Stress 149
  Vinegar can aid digestion 176
Dirty Dozen and Clean Fifteen List 76-77
Disconnected from food supply 41-42
Duped 15-32

Eat Now, Pay Later 27, 30
Eggs 123-128
  Action points 126-127
  American Heart Association 123
  Cholesterol (see cholesterol)
  Pasture-raised, organic 126
  Commercial 127
  Free range 127
  Omega 3 127
  Vegetarian 127
Emotional eating 55, 217
Environmental Protection Agency 72
Environmental Working Group (EWG) 71
Excess (see abundance)

Fahlberg, Constantine 96
Fats and oils 60, 103 - 108
  Action points 107-108
  Damaged oils 106
  Excess vegetable oil 104
  GM oils 104
  Purity 105-106
  Trans fats 105
Fermenting 63, 65, 100, 102, 149, 175
Fish and Seafood 129 - 130
  Action points 130
  Heavy Metals 130

Food and Drug Administration, FDA
  BPA and sippy cups 136
  GM safety 81
  Hormones in meat 114
  Sugar 92
  Sulphite 68
  Sweeteners 96
  Trans fats 105
Food Consciousness 195
Foundations for Change 190
Four Poisons of the Heart 170
Fructose 88, 90, 92
Fruit juice 90-92, 226
Generally recognized as safe (GRAS)
  Sweeteners 96
  Trans fats 106
GM/GMO 79-84
  Action Points
  Bt Corn 81
  Common commercial crops 79
  Monoculture 80
  Roundup Ready crops
  Safety 81
  Suicide (terminator) seeds 82
  vs. hybridization 79
  vs. Allah's variety 83
Gluten 100-102
Glyphosate
  Court case 33, 74
  in breakfast cereal (see cereal)
Grains 98 - 102
  Action points 77, 101-102
  Diabetes, and (see Diabetes)
  Fermenting, sprouting, soaking 100
  Gluten (see gluten)
  Pesticides 72, 100
  Wholegrain/refined/unrefined 99
  Wholegrain options 102
Gut 145 - 150
  Bacteria 145
  Digestion (see digestion)
  Dysbiosis 148
  Gut, food and mood 149
  Leaky gut 148
  Micribiome 145
  Pylori, Candida, SIBO 148
Health coaching/personal assessments 210-220

Heirloom plants and seeds 80-81, 83
High Fructose Corn Syrup (see additives)
Honey 93-94
  Action points 94
  Natural sweetener 97
  Healing food 152
  Natural food 174
  Eaten by the Prophet 176 -178, 221
Hormones (added to food)
  Meat 60, 113-114, 174
  Milk 60, 110
Hormones (in humans)
  Leptin resistence 56
  Stress 142, 197
How the Prophet Ate 172
  Bismillah 183
  Key to Healthy Eating 181
  Less frequency 187
  Mindfulness 182
  Natural Whole Food 174
  Sunnah of Eating 177-180
  Sunnah Foods 176-177
  Small Portions 185
How to eat an elephant 193
Hybrid, hybridization (see GM)

Ibn Al Qayyim
  Overeating 47
  Water 131
  Eating seasonal fruit 154
  Training ourselves 170
  Practice of the Prophet with food 175
Ikarians/Ikaria 155
Immune
  GM (see GM safety)
  Autoimmunity/Gluten (see Gluten)
  BPA (see BPA)
  PFCs 136
  Trauma 140
  Gut and, 147
Industrial Revolution 17
Infertility
  SAD/SMD Diet 17
  Pesticides 72
  GM 82
  BPA 135

Just one third 46-58
    Why it so hard 47-58

Key to healthy eating 36, 181, 192

Labels, beginner's guide 224-226
Langer, Ellen 21-22
Lawful and Unlawful 158-160
Leaky Gut (see gut health)
Leptin resistance (see hormones in humans)
Life overhaul, avoid 192-193

Mango, variety 83
Marketing (see Weapons of Mass Influence)
Mass Media 20
Mazur, Paul 18
Meat
    Action points 116-117
    Disconnected from food 53
    Excess consumption 37, 42, 53
    Environment 82, 114
    Ethics 115
    Hormones and pesticides 114
    Types of meat 113
    (Conventional, Organic, Processed)
Microbiome (see Gut)
Milk and dairy 109 - 111
    Action points 111
    Health food 109-110
    Hormones (see hormones in food)
Mind your language 198
Mindfulness 182-184
Monoculture (see GM)
Monsanto Bayer
    Glyphosate course case 33, 74
    Roundup Ready Seeds 81
    Terminator seeds 82
    Aspartame 96

Nafs 57, 187
Natural scarcity 154, 157, 175
Natural Whole Food 160, 174-175, 192, 194, 227
Neonicotinoid pesticides (see pesticides)
Neotame (see additives)
NSAIDS 148
NutraSweet (See Monsanto, Aspartame)
Nutrient density 58, 85
Oil and fats (see fats and oils)
Olive oil 104-105, 107, 176, 221

One third (see Just one third)

Packaging and cooking 135-136
    Action Points 136-137
    BPA (see BPA)
    PFCs 136
Paradox of Choice 43
Persistent Organic Pollutants 72-73
Pesticides
    Action points
        Fruit and veg 77
        Grains and legumes 77
        Meat 78
        Honey 78
    DDT 72
    Chlorpyrifos 73
    Dirty Dozen and Clean Fifteen 76
    Misleading research 74
    Neonicotinoids 73, 94
PFCs (Perfluorochemicals) 136
Portion Distortion 50
Predictably irrational 21
Processed food 17, 27, 34, 63
    Addicted 56
    Duped by design 51
    Nutritionally hungry 51
    SAD/SMD diet 17
Progress, not perfection 197
Propaganda 18-20
Public relations 18

Refined grains (see grains)
RSPCA 126

Sabido Effect 20
Sabido, Miguel 20
Saccharin (see additives)
Seasonal food 154-158
    Benefitts of seasonal/local 157
    Honey 93
    Natural whole food 174
    The Prophet: seasonal local 154
    S.O.U.L. food 184
Sedentary Lifestyle 29

Seeds
    Abundance 39

GM seeds and Roundup 81
   Heirloom variety 83
   Patented seeds 81
   Resource for heirloom seeds 81
   'Terminator' seeds 82
Serotonin 146
Shaitan 30
   Trickery 31
   Corruption 114
   Deception 168-169, 203
   Whispers 197
Simplemente Maria (see television)
Sleep (see total load)
Soaking (see grains)
Sprouting (see grains)
Standard American Diet (SAD) 16
Standard Modern Diet (SMD) 17
Stress (see total load)
Sucralose (see additives)
Sugar 88 - 92
   Action points 92
   Addiction 56, 91
   HFCS (see High Fructose Corn Syrup)
   Hidden sugar 89
   On labels 70
Sunnah of Eating (see how the Prophet ate)

Television
   Miguel Sabido (see Sabido, Miguel)
   Simplemente Maria 20-21
   Ven Conmigo (Come with Me) 20
The Creator Knows What the Creation
Needs 151-161
Then and Now, an overview 59-60
Torches of Freedom 19
Total Load 139 -
   Chemical Loaders 140
   Emotional/Spiritual Loaders 140
   Food Loaders 140
   General Physical Loaders 140
   Inhalant Loaders 141
   Lightening our load 142
TRANS Fats (see fats and oils)

Unrefined grains (see grains)

Ven Conmigo (Come with Me) - see
television

Vinegar
   Preserving 175
   Sunnah 176, 221
Vision of Health and Hope 33

Waste 44-46
Water 131
   Commodification of 132
   Purity 132
Weapons of mass influence
   scarcity 22
   social proof 23
   authority 23
   liking 23-24
   reciprocity 24
   consistency and comittment 24
Weekly delivery boxes 185
Whole Food Action Plan 227 - 228
Whole Food Shopping List 221
Whole Food Sources 185
Whole Grain Options 102
Wholegrains 102 (see grains)
World Health Organization (WHO)119

Yogurt 104, 107

Zero waste stores 185